Restart Your Recovery - 12 Things You Can Do To Get Back on the Beam

Recapturing Emotional Sobriety and Avoiding Relapse

by Taite Adams

Rapid   Response   Press
1730 Lighthouse Ter S, Ste 12

South   Pasadena,   FL   33707
www.rapidresponsepress.com

Ordering   Information:
Quantity sales. Special discounts are available on quantity purchases by corporations, associations, and others. For details, contact the publisher   at   the   address   above. Orders by U.S. trade bookstores and wholesalers. Please contact Rapid Response Press: Tel: (866) 983-3025; Fax: (855) 877-4736 or visit www. rapidresponsepress.com.

Printed in the United States of America

Publisher's   Cataloging-in-Publication   data
Adams,   Taite.
A title of a book : a subtitle of the same book / Taite Adams.
p.   cm.
ISBN   978-0-9889875-7-9
1. The main category of the book —Health —Other category. 2. Another subject category —Mind and Body. 3. More categories — Recovery.

Second Edition

==================

Limit of Liability/Disclaimer of Warranty

=================

Disclaimer

Disclaimer: This publication is designed to provide accurate and personal experience information in regard to the subject matter covered. It is sold with the understanding that the author, contributors, publisher are not engaged in rendering counseling or other professional services. If counseling advice or other expert assistance is required, the services of a competent professional person should be sought out.

==================

Medical Disclaimer

The information contained in this book is not intended to serve as a replacement for professional medical advice. Any use of the information in this book is at the reader's discretion. The author and publisher specifically disclaim any and all liability arising directly or indirectly from the use or application of any information contained in this book. A health care professional should be consulted regarding your specific situation.

To my Son - As motivators go, I couldn't have asked for a better, or cuter, one;

To Mom - For your love and support even when grossly undeserved;

To my Love - For the constant reminders of what living this program is really all about through your beautiful example and shining light.

Taite Adams

Get All The Books In The Series:

Kickstart Your Recovery - The Road Less Traveled to Freedom From Addiction

Safely Detox From Alcohol and Drugs at Home

Opiate Addiction - The Painkiller Addiction Epidemic, Heroin Addiction and The Way Out

Who is Molly? Molly Drug Facts, What is Ecstasy, and Life-Saving MDMA Effects Info

For More Information, visit http://www.taiteadams.com

Table of Contents

Taite Adams

Preface

I have several recovery-related books on the market and they are all born from my personal experiences. This one, however, is a bit more unique and resonates strongly with me for several reasons. One is that the experiences related are much more recent and another is that I believe this is something that is quite common in recovery yet isn't directly addressed as often as it should be.

The idea that we can stray from our recovery program isn't a new one. It happens all the time. Unfortunately, I believe that most people that move away from recovery are simply "written off" as it's assumed that they will probably go out and drink or do something else dreadful in very short order. In most cases, this is does come to pass. However, there are those of us who don't and who find that we simply aren't happy like we used to be, yet don't know how to get back on track. Ego, pride and simple stubbornness get in the way.

I found myself precisely in this place at 10 years sober and was in enough pain that I became willing to make some changes. I still knew, deep down, that drinking was not an option and years of recovery had given me an aversion to being in pain and in any sort of prolonged discomfort. I remembered that there was another way out and I had to make a start by asking for help. This is precisely what I did, among other things.

The list of 12 Things You Can Do to Get Back on the Beam are all Action items. We didn't think ourselves sober and aren't going to think or wish ourselves back into a place of serenity and peace. These are gifts from doing the work and I have found that simply making a beginning on each one of these items was all it took for the floodgates of recovery to open for me once again. If you or someone you love is in a slump in recovery, have moved completely away from the program, or have even gone back to active addiction, there is absolutely a way to get back on track and this book is for you.

What is Emotional Sobriety?

You can conquer others with power, but it takes true strength to conquer yourself. – Lao Tzu

I fear that there is a lot of confusion as to exactly what emotional sobriety is. Many people are under the impression that once we attain physical sobriety, through abstinence, and then continue to work a strong program, we should be happy, joyous and free all the live long day. We feel that there should be this perpetual pink cloud with a smattering of flying unicorns about, sprinkling the "blessings of the program" in our path. While the program does promise many blessings, this is not one of them.

Emotional sobriety has much more to do with balance and the ability to regulate one's emotions. There is an emotional intelligence that is developed as one continues to stay sober and works strong program. This involves staying in contact with other people in recovery, having a spiritual connection and remaining humble.

So, if you are feeling bad and going through a rough time does it mean that you don't have emotional sobriety? Not at all. Emotional sobriety is also about having the ability to feel one's feelings and to be in the present moment. When we get sober, we don't stuff things down anymore or hold onto resentments for months or years at a time. If we are still doing these sorts of things, therein lies the issue. A lack of emotional sobriety may show itself in such ways as the inability to regulate mood and behavior, not being able to gain perspective on feelings, inability to live in the present, and disturbances with close personal relationships.

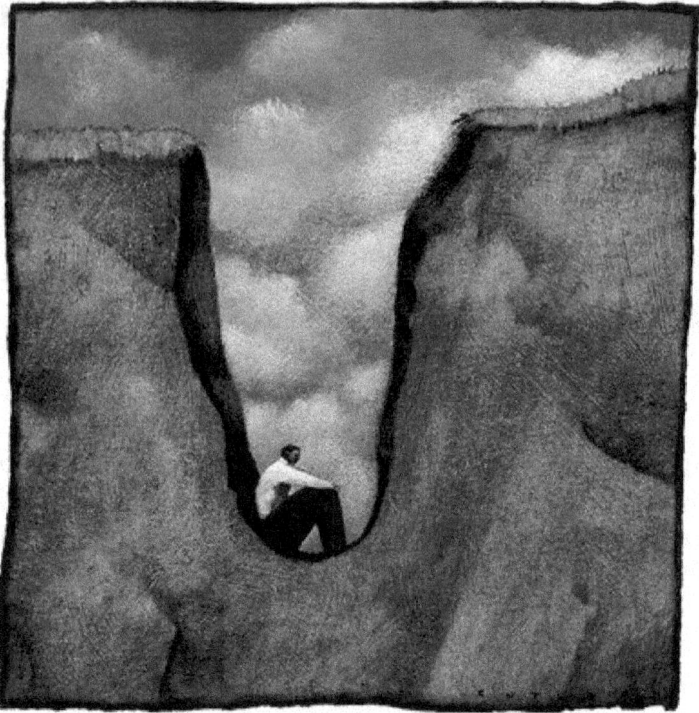

These are just a few ways to determine if emotional sobriety is a concern and, frankly, it's not a static thing. This is something that ebbs and flows with most of us. In fact, this continues to be an issue for many in recovery. In 1958, after over 20 years sober, AA co-founder Bill W realized that emotional sobriety was "the next frontier". He published a now famous article in The Grapevine magazine and was hopeful that AA members would make emotional sobriety an actual movement within the organization. This hasn't really happened but the topic continues to generate a lot of interest as so many in recovery start to get uncomfortable with where they're at and seek answers for avoiding relapse and recharging their programs.

Why Do We Move Away From Our Program?

Alcoholics are people who find something that works - and then stop doing it.

It's so common in recovery and in many people's stories, yet we still act shocked and dismayed when we find ourselves in such a situation. Whether you've picked up a drink or a drug or not, the realization that you've lost something in your recovery program can be a startling revelation. This usually happens gradually, though, over such a period of time that we hardly notice what is happening. One day, however, if we're lucky, we come to the realization that things just aren't right. We may feel a sense of dis-ease or discomfort, a profound loneliness, or creeping thoughts that perhaps a drink or a few pills would be a good idea. Regardless, if something isn't done - and soon - that path to destruction will find it's end and there is no telling whether or not we'll get another chance at recovery.

So, why do we move away from our recovery programs? There are a multitude of reasons but it all comes down to priorities. Remember, SLIP stands for Sobriety Loses Its Priority. Unless staying clean and sober and working a program remain at the top of the list, there is a danger of just this sort of thing happening. This actually happened to me at about 6 years sober. I was laid off from my corporate job and took that "opportunity" to start my own business. I made this my priority for the next 4 years. I cut out all of my service commitments, stopped working with a sponsor and cut my meetings to just one per week. As far as I was concerned, sobriety was still $\underline{A}$ priority but not the most important thing to me. As a result, my program suffered, my state of mind suffered and my overall health wasn't so hot either. At the end of those 4 years, I decide to make a change and Restart My Recovery. I saw that I was absolutely on the road to relapse if I did not take some massive action to get back on the beam.

What I have found during this process is an amazing renewal and a new appreciation for my recovery program and my emotional sobriety. I understand today that I don't have to pick up a drink in order to begin again in recovery. We can make a new beginning each day, by building on either the mistakes or victories of the past and find gratitude for all of it. Is it a tough road back? Sometimes it is - and it can be just like getting sober all over again. It can also be very renewing and a lot of fun if you are able to find that willingness once again. I think that many of us hit emotional bottoms in recovery that we can use as motivators for the actions that need to be taken for further spiritual progress and growth. If you've found that you've hit one of these, you may be ready to Restart Your Recovery.

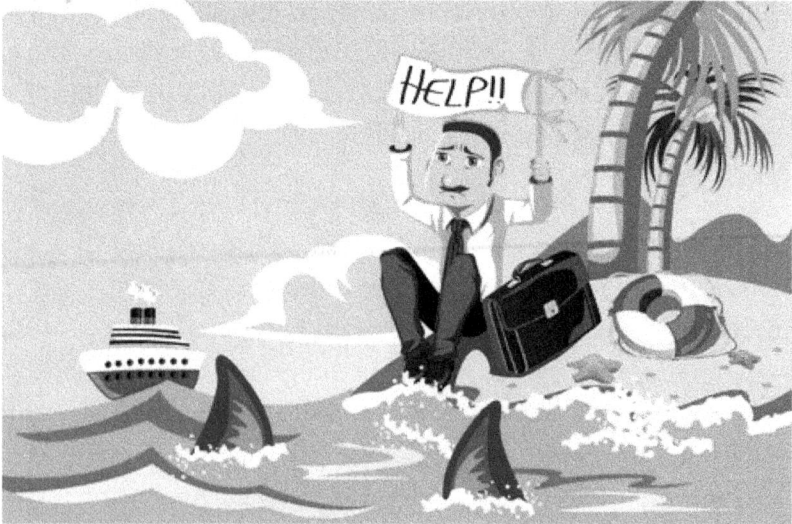

Your present circumstances don't determine where you can go; they merely determine where you start. -Nido Qubein

Signs of Relapse

I don't need help quitting, I have quite a thousand times! I need help STAYING QUIT! - The White Book

If you are thinking about Restarting Your Recovery, the assumption is that you have had recovery before. Think for a minute about the stages through which that came to pass. In essence, we get sober Physically first, when we put down the drink or drug, then Mentally/Emotionally when our thoughts start clearing up and then Spiritually through working a program. When we lose our sobriety, the exact opposite happens. Spirituality slips away first. We stop relying on a higher power and take back control. Then, the Mental/Emotional aspect of recovery begins chipping away. Finally, the Physical is final stage where we again pick up a drink or a drug to ease the pain and discomfort that we are feeling. This can be a very long process yet somewhere in the middle is where things start to get very uncomfortable and many of us find that we're in enough pain to make a change.

Because relapse is a process, and can be a long one, there are many opportunities along the way to use new ways of thinking and new actions to reverse the process, regain emotional sobriety and avoid relapse. So, before we get into what you can do to reverse the process and "get back on the beam", a basic understanding of the stages of relapse may be in order. In 1982, researchers Terence T. Gorski and Merlene Miller identified a set of warning signs or steps that typically lead up to a relapse. Over the years, additional research has confirmed that the steps described in the Gorski and Miller study are "reliable and valid" predictors of alcohol and drug relapses. Here they are in a nutshell:

- **Change in Attitude** - This goes along the same lines of a shift in priorities, wherein you decide that recovery just isn't as important as it used to be. There may a return of some old attitudes and ideas, sometimes referred to as "stinking thinking".

- **Elevated Stress** - An increase in stress can be due to major life events or a broken shoe lace. The danger in over-reacting to normal everyday situations is high as well as the tendency to have mood swings.

- **Reactivation of Denial** - This isn't about you having a disease. It's about you being able to manage your life and your addiction on your own. You may be scare or worried but dismiss these feelings and stop sharing with others.

- **Recurrence of Postacute Withdrawal Symptoms** - Anxiety, depression, memory loss and sleep problems can continue long after you stop drinking and using, and these symptoms can return in times of high stress. The danger is the temptation to self-medicate to alleviate them.

- **Behavior Change** - In early sobriety you may have developed some healthy habits that replaced your compulsive behaviors. Slow abandonment of these habits is common, as well as poor judgment and return to more impulsive behavior.

- **Social Breakdown** - You begin to isolate, stop hanging around sober friends and withdraw from family members. You may cut way back on meetings or stop attending them altogether, making excuses to be alone.

- **Loss of Structure** - Abandonment of daily routine that was established in sobriety. You may sleep late, ignore personal hygiene or skip meals. You may begin focusing on one small part of life to the exclusion of everything else.

- **Loss of Judgment** - You begin to have trouble making decisions or you make unhealthy decisions. Managing feelings and emotions may become difficult and you may become confused easily. You may also become annoyed or angry easily.

- **Loss of Control** - You make irrational choices and are unable to interrupt or alter those choices. You begin to actively cut off people who can help you and lose confidence in your ability to manage your life. You begin to think that you can drink socially or use drugs recreationally and can control it.

- **Loss of Options** - You begin limiting your options by stopping attending all meetings and any therapy. You may feel angry, lonely, frustrated, and resentful. You might feel helpless and desperate and come to believe that there are only three ways out: insanity, suicide or self-medication with alcohol and drugs.

- **Relapse** - You attempt controlled, "social" or short-term alcohol or drug use, but are disappointed at the results and experience guilt and shame. You lose control quickly and are out of control. This causes more problems with relationships, jobs, money, mental and physical health. You need help getting sober again.

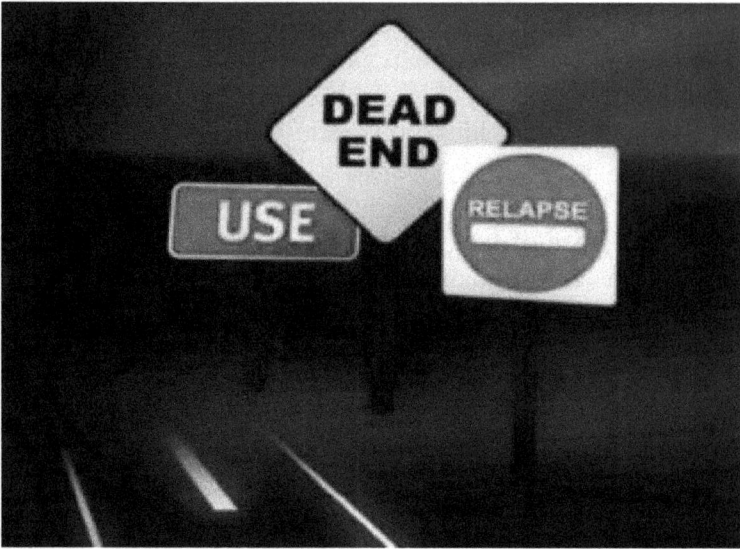

If that process isn't "sobering", I don't know what is. I was able to recognize a lot of things in that list that were going on with me during those 4 years that I moved away from the program. The most important thing to take away from this, however, is that this is a process that can be stopped if you are able to recognize what is going on and are willing to make a change. If you aren't, picking up again is an inevitability in my opinion and that just compounds the misery and the return, IF I am even given another chance at it. So, if you have reached one of those emotional bottoms, see yourself somewhere on this relapse continuum (ie - crazy train) and want to get off, or have picked up and want to get back on track, you can Restart Your Recovery and get back on the beam today by doing the following actions.

The best way out is always through. —Robert Frost

1 - Go Back to Meetings

If we don't change our direction, we are likely to end up where we are headed.
-Ancient Chinese Proverb

This can be hard, or not, depending on your circumstances. Pride is a cunning thing and our disease uses this to keep us isolated and sick. It's not always easy for an alcoholic or addict to return to their home group after a period of absence and admit that they really need those guys after all. What generally happens, though, is that everyone is thrilled that you're back, that you're safe and that you want to try something different. Many people will be more than eager to share their own stories of life away from meetings with you and what brought them back into the fold.

Depending on where you live or on how long you've been away from meetings, there may not be a lot of familiar faces. That's fine also. One important thing is to let people know where you're at and what you're doing. My experience was somewhere in the middle of this. I had lived in the same area for over 5 years but didn't really have many recovery connections there or have a home group. I returned to meetings daily in a place that I had been before but really didn't know anyone on a personal level. I did speak up, however, and let people know who I was and what I was doing. It wasn't easy but it was worth it. I made some new friends pretty quickly and set to work establishing the solid support system that I had been lacking for so many years.

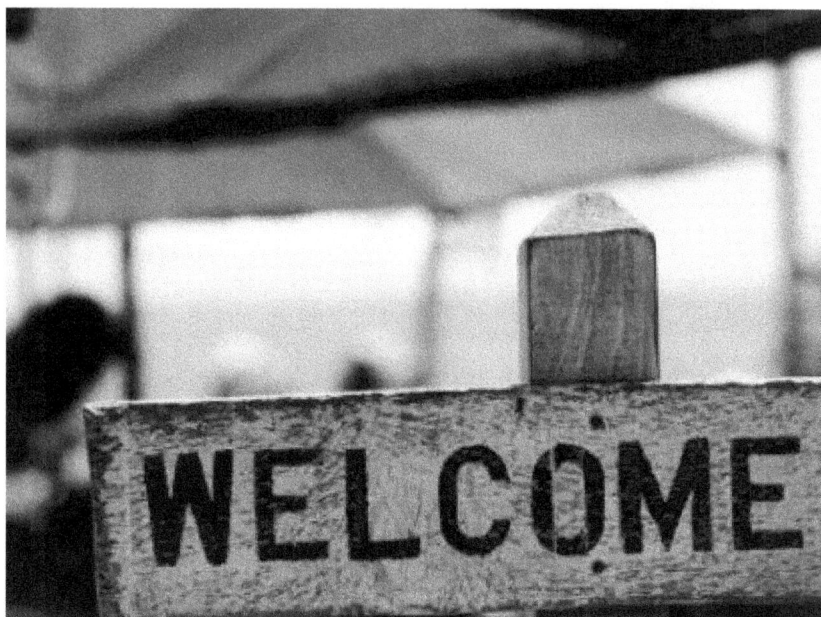

Separate reeds are easily broken; but bound together they are strong and hard to break apart. -The Midrash

Commit to a New 90 in 90

Be miserable. Or motivate yourself. Whatever has to be done, it's always your choice. -Wayne Dyer

Newcomers are often horrified when they are first told that they should do 90 meetings in 90 days. However, there are valid reasons for this and many people with time in recovery often "re-up" and commit to doing another 90 in 90. This is commonplace when moving to a new area, in order to establish a new routine and support system and is very appropriate when we are talking about making a new start in recovery and working on emotional sobriety, regardless of where you are and who you "already know".

So, why the 90 in 90 anyway? Why not 60 in 60? Well, the 90-day point actually represents a sort of threshold, first in clearing away the effects of drugs and alcohol but also in setting new habits. A recent Time Magazine article states *"... It turns out that this is just about how long it takes for the brain to reset itself and shake off the immediate influence of a drug. Researchers at Yale University have documented what they call the sleeper effect--a gradual re-engaging of proper decision making and analytical functions in the brain's prefrontal cortex--after an addict has abstained for at least 90 days."* There are many benefits to, number one - taking suggestions and number two - actually doing the 90 meetings in 90 days.

A big part of this is the willingness to take the suggestion and make the commitment to change your life for the better, which is the whole idea. Another benefit is the exposure to a continuity of meetings that will allow you to meet some new people and get some support. This ensures that the program once again becomes a priority, which can be a great confidence and self-esteem boost as you are keeping a daily commitment. I am essentially a creature of habit. I had gotten into the unhealthy habit for several years of staying home alone. I needed to change that habit by committing to meetings again and doing 90 meetings in 90 days was a great start.

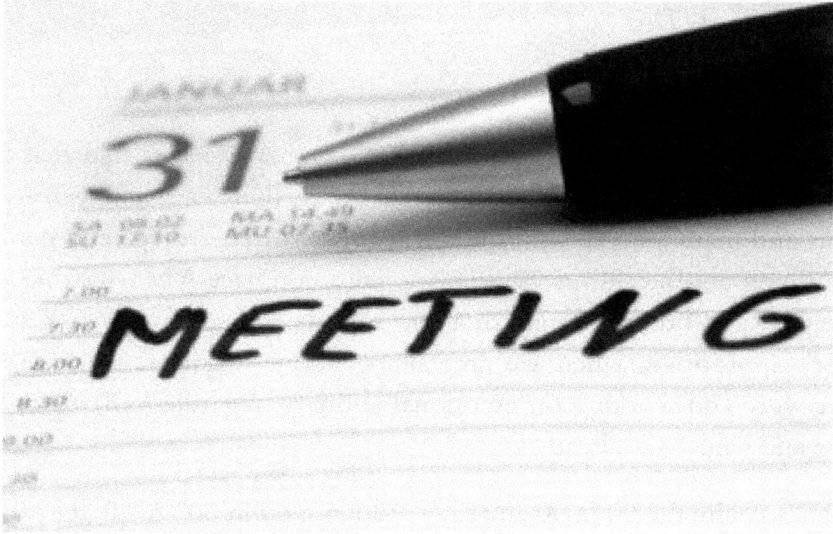

Try Some New Meetings

If you want what you've never had, you must do what you've never done.

I can't begin to count the number of times I've heard people talk about how they stopped going to meetings because they "got sick of AA". If you can relate to this, you're not alone. However, I urge you to go back to the third chapter and look at the relapse process. You'll see on there that moving away from social circles and support groups is actually about halfway down, so the there was a lot going on internally that we weren't dealing with prior to us "getting sick of AA" and walking away. Regardless, many a new meeting have sprung up courtesy of a resentment and a coffee pot, so that is always another option. If you don't want to return to your home group or start your own meeting, consider trying out some different meetings in your area.

Depending on where you live, this may be a simple prospect or not. Where I live, there are over 110 meetings per day in the county and one could go to a different meeting each day for a year. In fact, I became "bored" just a few years into sobriety and started checking off meetings on my "Where and When" as I drove around and visited new meetings in the area, determined to visit them all at some point. I didn't, but it was a fun project. If you live in a more rural area, I am sure that there are still a few meetings that you haven't frequented and could perhaps give a try. One thing to keep in mind, however, is that you'll want to have some sort of consistency about your meetings as you get back into the program and Restart Your Recovery. You'll need to give people a chance to get to know you and going to an entirely different meeting, with different people, everyday isn't going to do that.

If you don't currently have a home group, use this opportunity to figure out which meeting you are most comfortable at and get one. This group becomes your "home base", if you will, and will be the meeting that you make a commitment to attend as often as you are able. An advantage of being a member of a Home Group and attending regularly is that you have a group of people who really get to know you well and become "invested" in your life and your trials. They will visit you in the hospital, call when you lose a loved one and offer advice when you ask them for it. Sounds a bit corny reading it but it's comforting as heck when you need these people and it's actually quite nice to be able to be there for them as well. The key to all of this is simply make a start and get your butt back to meetings, plain and simple.

A.A. is no success story in the ordinary sense of the word. It is a story of suffering transmuted, under grace, into spiritual progress. AS BILL SEES IT, p. 35

2 - Get a Service Commitment

. . . he has struck something better than gold. . . . He may not see at once that he has barely scratched a limitless lode which will pay dividends only if he mines it for the rest of his life and insists on giving away the entire product.
ALCOHOLICS ANONYMOUS, p. 129

Of course we hear in the rooms all the time that "we have to give it away in order to keep it". This is absolutely true, yet there are few actions that you can take like this that will give you the overwhelming sense of peace and belonging. Service work is always done with no hope of reward or praise, with only the idea that by helping someone else in recovery, both people are benefiting. Though there is plenty of debate about what works and what doesn't with regards to recovery, there is little disputing that helping others who have drug or alcohol addiction problems can be very helpful to one's own recovery. There is a saying that many in recovery circles repeat that goes, "When I got busy, I got better." What it means is, in their effort to maintain sobriety, they found that doing service work to help others actually helped them stay clean and sober. In fact, numerous studies have provided evidence to this effect.

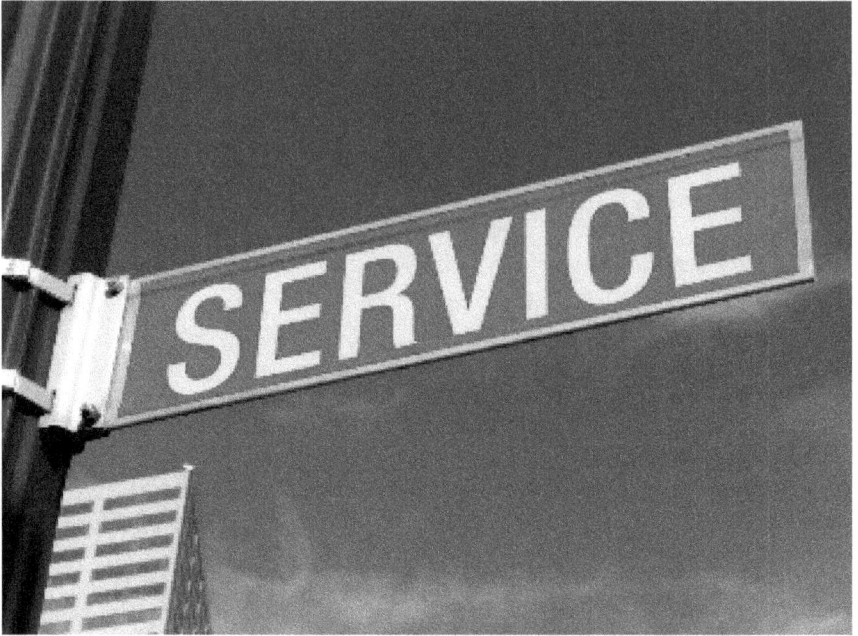

In a 2004 survey published in the Journal of Drug and Alcohol Abuse, alcohol addiction researcher Sarah Zenmore reported that giving support helped recovering alcoholics and addicts to maintain their sobriety. "Studies have shown that AA involvement is a strong predictor of sustained recovery," she reported. That included "meeting attendance as well as helping activities such as doing service in the AA fellowship and being a sponsor."

Maria E. Pagano, PhD, of Case Western Reserve University School of Medicine, in a published review cited several empirical studies that support the "helper therapy principle" or the idea that when someone helps another person with a similar condition, they help themselves. Dr. Pagano and colleagues evaluated the decade long of treatment outcomes using data from a single site in Project MATCH, the largest multi-site randomized clinical trial on behavioral treatments of alcoholism sponsored by the National Institute on Alcohol Abuse and Alcoholism. Results showed that participation in Alcoholics

Anonymous-related Helping (AAH) produced lowered alcohol use and increased interest in others at each subsequent follow-up assessment. "The AAH findings suggest the importance of getting active in service, which can be in a committed 2-month AA service position or as simple as sharing one's personal experience in recovery to another fellow sufferer." This study also found that alcoholics engaged in AAH did more step-work and attended more meetings than those not helping others.

Helping other people in recovery is one of the most effective ways to stay motivated. It reminds people in recovery about where they have come from, and what they would be going back to if they ever relapsed. Interested in avoiding relapse? Don't avoid service work! Also, alcoholics have a tendency to be very self-absorbed. By thinking about and helping others, this allows them to take the focus off of themselves and get a change in perspective. Helping others also helps to continue to build self-esteem as the giver feels that they are giving something back to society. Of key importance here, however, is that by helping other people stay sober, the individual continues to strengthen their own recovery. Not sure where to start? There are many opportunities for service work in AA, NA and other recovery groups.

Make yourself a blessing to someone. Your kind smile or pat on the back just might pull someone back from the edge. -Carmelita Elliott

Service to a Home Group

The only ones among you who will be really happy are those who will have sought and found how to serve. -*Albert Schweitzer*

The idea of doing Service Work can sound very ominous and scary, even for some of us that have been around the program for awhile. It's not at all and can be as simple as doing a few things for your home group. Remember, Groups like Alcoholics Anonymous could not function without the voluntary services provided by its members and that coffee that you're drinking at the meeting doesn't make itself. If you wish to make a small start in service and don't know where to begin, simply ask. There are plenty of opportunities at the group level to be of service. Here are just a few examples:

- Making coffee at a meeting
- Serving as official "greeter" at a meeting
- Helping to set up before or clean up after a meeting
- Welcoming newcomers
- Chairing or sharing at a meeting
- Give rides to and from meetings to members that need them
- Taking an official service role within a recovery group, for example treasurer or secretary
- Making time to speak to people who are obviously struggling with addiction problems

As you can see, none of these are real "time killers" and you will get back so much more than you give. Giving back is a huge confidence and self esteem booster and this is something that many of us need as we are repaving our path in recovery. In fact those people who devote some time to helping others are less likely to suffer from depression and helping others in recovery serves to remind us where we came from. Once you get your feet wet at the Group Level again, you may wish to consider other service commitments to the organization.

Service to Intergroup, District and Area

Your job now is to be at the place where you may be of maximum helpfulness to others; so never hesitate to go anywhere if you can be helpful. -AA, 2001, p. 102

Before I took my 4 year hiatus from recovery, I was very involved in service work. In fact, I was entrenched from the beginning. I remember telling my story at a new meeting (to me) at about a year sober. A lady walked up to me after the meeting and said "This is your new home group and you are our new Secretary". I just smiled and said "OK". From there I became a GSR (General Service Representative), then a DCM (District Committee Member), then a District Committee Chairperson and then on to an Area Committee Chairperson over the next 5 years. It was an amazing learning experience and made me feel like an important little cog in a very massive global recovery wheel. I traveled to a lot of Area meetings, met new people and learned about the Traditions, the history of AA and about myself. However, when I started my own business I made the choice to walk away from that service work and its small time commitment. This was a mistake. Service to AA on this level is important and rewarding, if you can do it, and can be done in many different ways.

The Twelve Traditions of Alcoholics Anonymous (you can apply the same to NA and other 12-step Fellowships) make clear the principle that A.A., as such, should never be organized, that there are no bosses and no government in A.A. Yet at the same time, the Traditions recognize the need for some kind of organization to carry the message in ways that are impossible for the local groups - such as publication of uniform literature and public information resources, helping new groups get started, publishing an international magazine, and carrying the message in other languages into other countries. The Conference structure of A.A. is the framework in which these "general services" are carried out. It is a method by which A.A.'s collective group conscience can speak forcefully and put its desires for worldwide services into effect. It is the structure that takes the place of government in A.A., ensuring that the full voice of A.A. will be heard and guaranteeing that movement-wide services will continue to function under all conditions.

Today, general services include all kinds of activities within the Conference structure, carried on by districts, area committees, delegates, trustees, the General Service Office and the Grapevine (A.A.'s monthly magazine). Usually, these services affect A.A. as a whole. A.A. has been called an upside-down organization because by looking at an organizational chart the A.A. group or meeting is on top and "headquarters" is on the bottom.

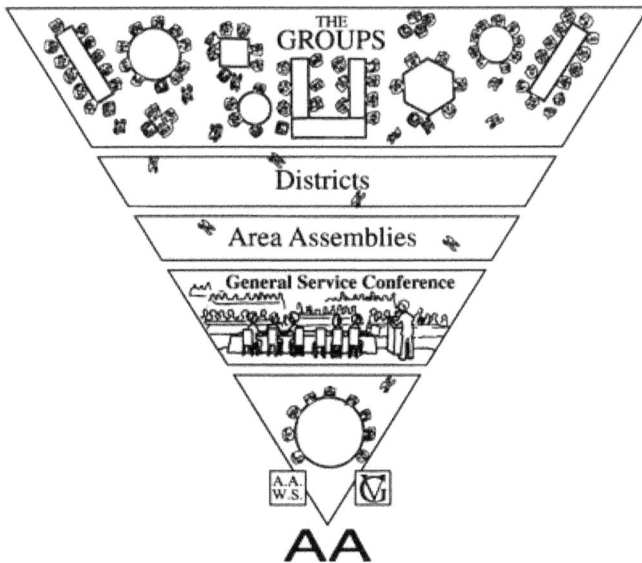

THE GROUPS

Districts

Area Assemblies

General Service Conference

A.A. W.S.

AA

There are so many opportunities for service work at the Intergroup, District and Area level that it would take pages to list them all. Suffice it to say, there is a service job out there waiting for you should you have the willingness, and a little time, to take it on. However, here are a few examples of some of the things that you could do:

- Visiting substance abusers in local jails and in prison
- Taking telephone calls from addicts looking for help
- Talk to the public or professionals about addiction
- Take meetings into local treatment centers
- Preserve and pass on the history of AA
- Help people with Special Needs get to meetings
- Work on an AA website committee
- Represent your Home Group at Intergroup, District or Area
- Represent your District at the Area Level

- Service to the Area through Committees and elected offices

As you can see, there are plenty of opportunities here, and should you do a little research, you will likely find many positions sadly "vacant" for lack of a willing "servant". Service work is the opportunity for recovery to become more than just about oneself. It provides the opportunity to take those things that we learn as recovering addicts and alcoholics and move further away from the isolation of the addiction and become involved with helping others in the program.

The Promises tell us that we will lose interest in selfish things and gain interest in our fellows and that self-seeking will slip away. This is an important part of the transition to service work. Finally, it becomes more important to take what we have learned from the program and to begin to give back. All of this is another exercise in establishing new behaviors that will be incompatible with addictive behavior. One cannot stay sober on service work alone, however. There are always more positive actions that need be taken.

3 - Re-Work the Steps

I have found that the process of discovering who I really am begins with knowing who I really don't want to be. — *Alcoholics Anonymous*

I say "Re-work the steps" as the assumption is that, if you have had some time in recovery, that you have done this before. This may not necessarily be the case. In fact, I've known people with years in recovery who have NEVER worked the steps. I also know several people who have many years in the program, yet didn't work the steps until they were in the program for quite some time, say 5 or more years. Some of you can probably relate to this and others are probably scratching your heads and wondering why in the world anyone would do that? I personally worked the steps with a sponsor in the first year of sobriety but I do understand how this situation could come about.

Some people are able to maintain abstinence from alcohol and drugs with the help of meetings and the fellowship. This is not to say, however, that they have found any sort of quality sobriety and doubtful much serenity or true happiness, ie- emotional sobriety. This is why many people do, at some point, decide to make a change and work the steps. When I first got sober, I was told that "the same person that walked through those doors will drink again" and I believed this to be true so I took all of the suggestions, which included getting a sponsor and working the steps. I have actually worked the steps with a sponsor several times since and highly recommend it to anyone who is making a new start in recovery and looking for ways to avoid relapse.

The recovery "Program" of AA itself is the 12 Steps. What working the 12 Steps does is allow us to take a look at the role our ego and pride has played in our lives, particularly in our addictions and our actions. The personal reflection that takes place and confession actually helps to establish new levels of self awareness and helps to overcome the shame that nearly all of us have, whether we are initially aware of it or not. Scientists believe that this process may actually help to "rewire the brain" in that the pre-frontal cortex is reinvigorated. Our sense of self is impacted profoundly by the process of making amends, that also serves to alleviate feelings of guilt and limit stressors that could trigger relapse. Finally, and certainly not least, there is a renewed spiritual connection that takes place through this entire process. This is, of course, very difficult to measure but there is no doubt that this is an essential element to, and byproduct of, working the Steps.

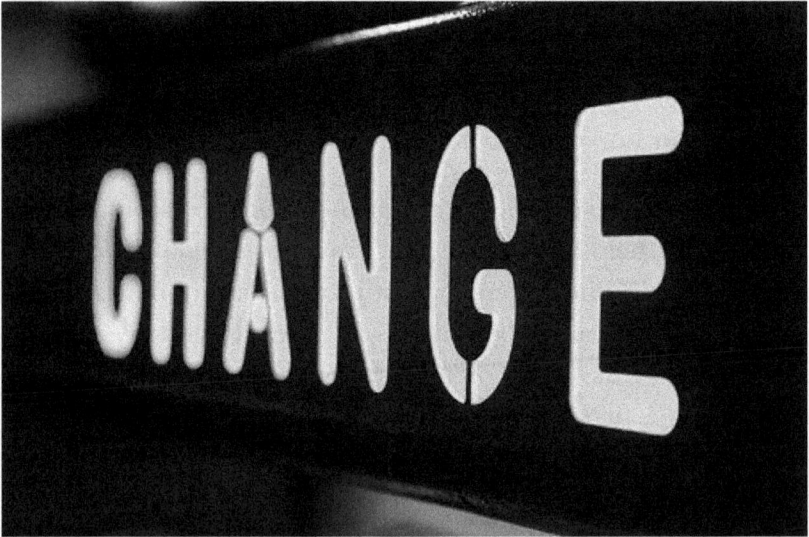

If we don't change, we don't grow. If we don't grow, we aren't really living. - Gail Sheehy

Use Your Sponsor

There were deep secrets, hidden in my heart, never said for fear others would scoff or snear. At last I can reveal my sufferings, for the strength I once felt in silence has lost all it's power. -Deidra Sarault

A large part of working the steps, obviously, is contact and working closely with your sponsor. Don't think for one second that you are the first person ever to have stopped calling their sponsor and, perhaps in their eyes, to have dropped off the face of the earth. Again, our pride wants to keep us isolated and doesn't want us to pick up that phone and "make contact" with each other. The reality is, if you do have a sponsor and have neglected the relationship for a period of time, they have probably been concerned about you and will be thrilled to hear from you. This should be one of your first stops in re-establishing your program. Give them a call or talk to them after a meeting - don't shoot them a text or an email.

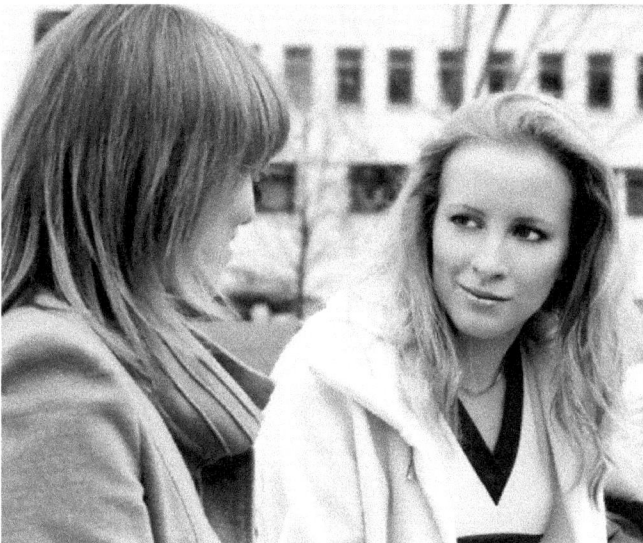

Get together with your sponsor and be honest about where you're at and what has been going on with you. Let them know that you are making a new start in recovery and would like to Rework the steps with them. Also ask for any other "suggestions" that they may have for you on this journey, which may include attending certain meetings, doing service work, reading some literature or calling them on a regular basis. If it all sounds like "getting back to basics", that's great. Because, it is!

Get a New Sponsor if Needed

. . . what comes to us alone may be garbled by our own rationalization and wishful thinking. The benefit of talking to another person is that we can get his direct comment and counsel on our situation. . . . TWELVE STEPS AND TWELVE TRADITIONS, p. 60

Sponsor - sponsee relationships are all different and many times we are given what we need at just the right time in our recovery. Sometimes, however, relationships and circumstances change and these relationships are no longer mutually beneficial. It may also be possible that your sponsor has moved away, passed away or is having their own struggles with life and sobriety. These are all valid reasons for finding a new sponsor. Here are some unreasonable motives for changing sponsors just so we're clear:

- Wanting to have a more popular sponsor.
- Choosing a new sponsor because they are more attractive.
- Changing sponsors in the hope of getting financial or employment help from this other individual.
- Leaving their current sponsor because they don't like being challenged in any way.
- Changing for the sake of change is not a good reason. It can take a bit of time to develop a good relationship with a sponsor and regularly changing their sponsor may mean never enjoying such a relationship.
- Some people want to find a new sponsor because they've had a minor argument with their current one. It is usually best to work these things out, or the individual will develop the habit of always running away.

- Some people will have expectations of sponsors that are unrealistically high. This means that they will be searching for a relationship that doesn't exist.

If you do need to end the relationship with a current sponsor, do so face to face if at all possible and with the utmost respect. Simply thank them for all of their help and let them know that you are going to be working with someone else in the future. That's it. If you are faced with getting a new sponsor, or one for the first time ever, and are not sure what to look for, here is a brief reminder:

- Generally has more years of sobriety than you (there are exceptions to this rule)
- The same gender as you (there are exceptions to this rule also)
- Emphasizes the Steps and Traditions of the Program
- Has what we want in terms of recovery, serenity and emotional sobriety

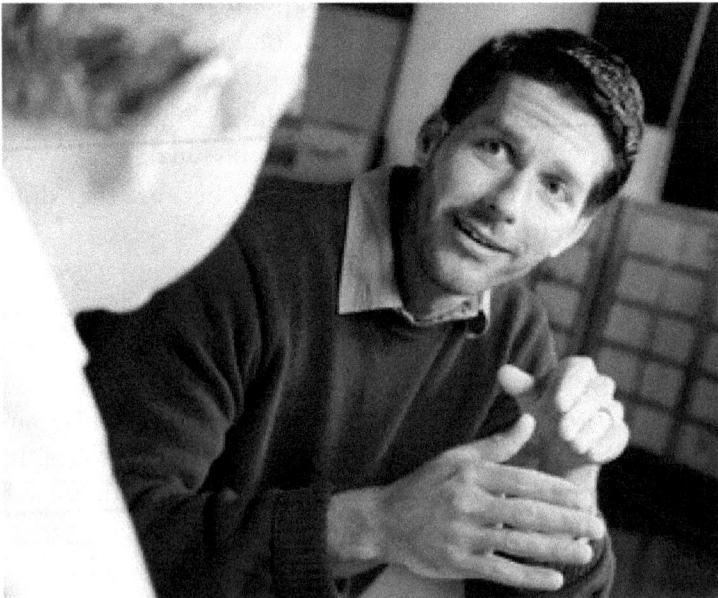

These are just some basic guidelines to use in your search. I could list a slew of them that would just serve to bog you down and ensure that you never find anyone to fit the bill. Remember, these are other "human beings", not saints. What we are looking for is someone who is successfully working a recovery program and is willing to help you do the same. If you get stuck here, don't be afraid to ask group members for help and suggestions. Essentially, look for someone who's recovery inspires you and ask them if they would be willing to be your sponsor. It's that simple.

4 - Work With Newcomers

The dark past is the greatest possession you have — the key to life and happiness for others. With it you can avert death and misery for them. -Alcoholics Anonymous, p. 124

Newcomers are vitally important to the AA program and work with newcomers should be an essential part of a well-rounded recovery program. "The newcomer is the most important person in the room" - Heard this one before?   Consider the famous picture of the "The Man on the Bed", who is representative of AA #3, Bill D.   Bill D had been trying to get sober. He had been medically detoxed six times in less than a year. Religion – that didn't work. He was a deacon at his church. He was the classic one who believed in God but was quite sure God did not believe in him.

At the same time, Bob and Bill were desperately trying to stay sober themselves. They knew their sobriety depended on talking to another suffering alcoholic. According to Ernie Kurtz in his history of AA, "Not God," Mrs. D told her alcohol-poisoned husband, "part of the plan these two drunks had for staying sober themselves was to tell their plan to another drunk: that was how they were going to stay sober." Later Bill D would reflect, "All the other people that had talked to me wanted to help me, and my pride prevented me from listening to them, and caused only resentment on my part, but I felt as if I would be a real stinker if I did not listen to a couple of fellows for a short time, if that would cure them."

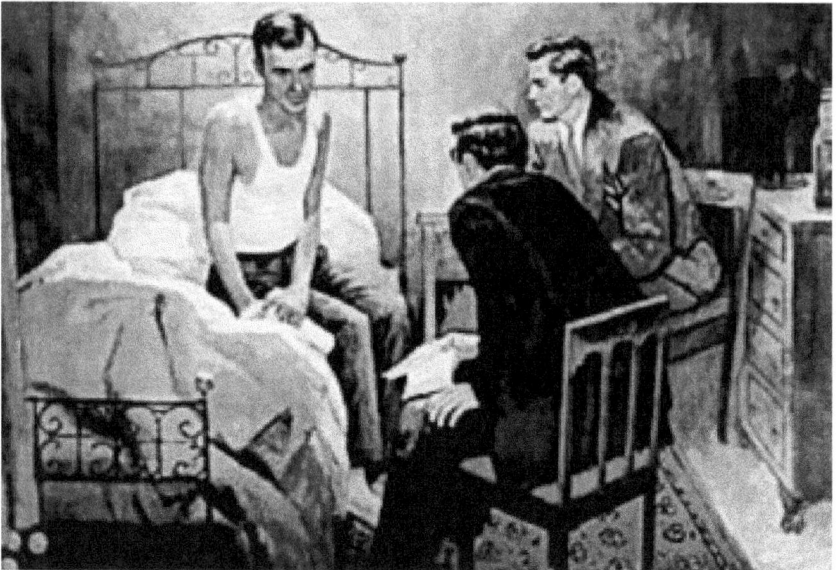

So Bill D let the first two AA members help him, for their own good initially. Only later did he realize that these two could help him; they had been where he had been, felt what he had felt and experienced that overwhelming despair that only another alcoholic can describe. But these drunks were sober. Maybe, just maybe, he could stay sober too.

And so it goes. Sharing our experience, strength and hope with those new in the program enables them to identify with us and this is where we find our common ground in recovery that allows us to be able to move forward and work together with a new level of trust. It is commonly said that "one should never say 'No' to AA" and this is meant in the context of doing service work, including sponsorship, if you are able. Volunteering, especially with the newly sober, reminds you where you've been and can easily return to again if you pick up a drink or drug. This is relapse prevention at its finest. It's impossible to be self-centered, I was told, while working on behalf of others.

If you are worried about how to be a good sponsor, don't. First, be assured that this is a very common fear and, if you have had a good sponsor or two on your journey, you really already know how to be one. However, here are just a few factors to consider when working with newcomers:

- **Be patient**: Many times, newcomers don't fully understand the scope of work involved in the 12 steps, and may find themselves getting impatient. Sometimes we want to rush through the steps or have a mental timetable as to when they should be complete. My first sponsor was methodical and patient when explaining what the steps involved, and gave me much more reasonable expectations.
- **Be available**: Being a sponsor means being able to be reached by your sponsees throughout the day, as well as at odd and random hours. Recovery isn't easy, nor is it predictable or timely. Make sure your sponsee has all of your contact information, and respond to them when you can. If you can't take their call or email right away, get back to them as soon as possible.
- **Be knowledgeable**: Make sure to keep current with all of the literature relevant to your recovery group in order to give your sponsee a more well-rounded picture of what's going on in the world of recovery. Stay active in both Big Book and Step and Traditions meetings.
- **Have a sponsor**: Just because you are a sponsor doesn't mean you shouldn't keep yours. Sponsors are human like anyone else, and need a shoulder to cry on or an ear to bend, often frequently. By having a sponsor to help you maintain your focus and keep you grounded, you can do the same for your sponsee.

Being a good sponsor is a challenge, but it also can help you in your own recovery. By helping others go through the steps of recovery, you can help fortify the steps and their meanings in your own life and your own recovery.

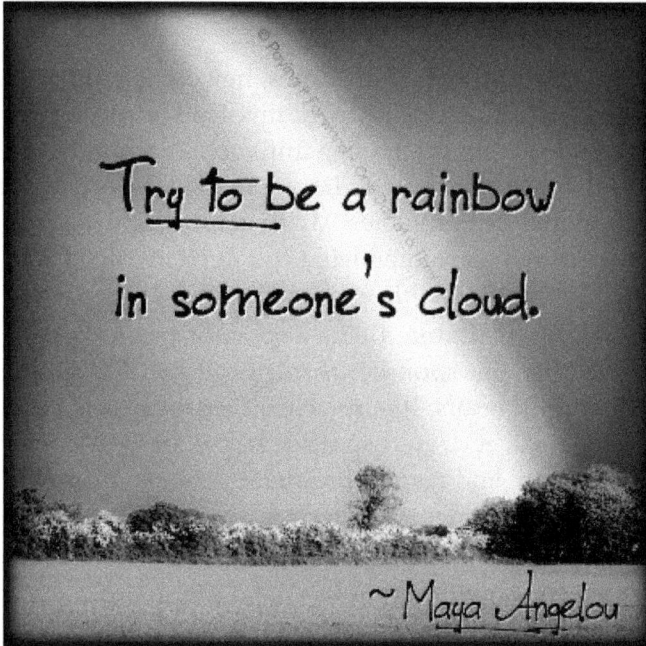

Life will take on new meaning. To watch people recover, to see them help others, to watch loneliness vanish, to see a fellowship grow up about you, to have a host of friends— this is an experience you must not miss. We know you will not want to miss it. Frequent contact with newcomers and with each other is the bright spot of our lives. ALCOHOLICS ANONYMOUS, p. 89

5 - Get Involved in the Fellowship

Give freely of what you find and join us. We shall be with you in the Fellowship of the Spirit, and you will surely meet some of us as you trudge the Road of Happy Destiny. —*Alcoholics Anonymous, page 164*

Many people get bogged down in the difference between a 12 Step Program and the Fellowship. It's not that difficult to distinguish which is which. The program of Alcoholics Anonymous, for example, is everything between the covers of the Big Book and the 12 and 12, which explains how we use and apply the 12 Steps to our lives. Yet, the Program cannot exist without the Fellowship, which are active and participating members of the groups who share their experience, strength and hope with each other. Fellowship is happening during meetings, yet it is also happening when "any two or more of us gather to share our experience, strength and hope". This could be over coffee, dinner, a game of golf or a day on the lake.

Reading, or hearing this, many people also seem to think that simply going to meeting is "enough". It may be enough to stay sober for many people but there is so much more available by getting involved in the Fellowship and it doesn't take a lot of effort to do it and reap the rewards.

Friendship of a kind that cannot easily be replaced tomorrow must have its roots in common interests and shared beliefs. -Barbara W. Tuchman

Go to Dinner, Coffee, Picnics, Banquets...

The feeling of having shared in a common peril is one element in the powerful cement which binds us. — Alcoholics Anonymous

I consider myself to be a loner - still. I was raised an only child and became accustomed, and very comfortable, being alone. I still find it to be against my nature to be in groups of people or at large gatherings. However, when I came into AA many years ago, I was told that I needed to "get into the middle of the Program", meet people and start "hanging out", so I did this. I didn't like it, but I did it. I showed up a meetings early and slowly got to know some people and started going out to dinner afterwards some nights. I also met groups that liked to do things together on the weekends so always had people to go to the beach or camping with. This was Fellowship at its finest.

Then I moved to another area and didn't "get into the middle of the Program" there. I did my alone thing and sobriety wasn't my priority for several years. As a result, I didn't really have many people that I felt I could call if I needed to chat, though I'm sure this isn't true. I simply felt disconnected yet convinced myself that I was perfectly comfortable and "ok" in that place. The truth was that I needed that Fellowship in my life in order to maintain my emotional sobriety and to continue to grow. So, when I decided to Restart my recovery, I knew that the Fellowship had to be a big part of that.

When I did return to meetings and let people know who I was, what was going on with me and what I was trying to do, I simply had to remain willing and open. People immediately came up to me and started inviting me out to dinner after the meeting. I started going - even though my instinct was to run back home. I made some great new friends in a very short time and my support group just keeps growing and getting stronger. These are people that I see and talk to outside of meetings and that I have allowed to get to know me. I know that they would be there for me should I need them and they know the same of me. That's what the Fellowship is all about and it doesn't take a lot of effort to get started. Most districts have plenty of AA-related Fellowship opportunities such as Group Picnics and Founder's Day Banquets, but the unofficial "coffee after the meeting" is all it takes to make a start.

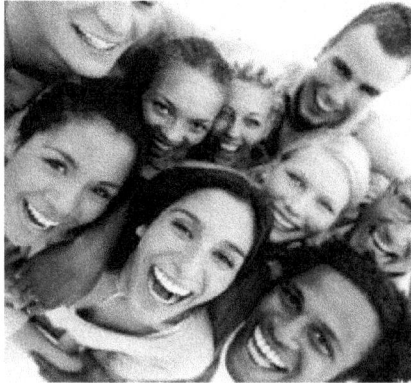

The average person living to age 70 has 613, 000 hours of life. This is too long a period not to have fun.

6 - Attend AA Workshops, Roundups and Conventions

. . . no society of men and women ever had a more urgent need *for continuous effectiveness and permanent unity. We alcoholics see that we must work together and hang together, else most of us will finally die alone.* ALCOHOLICS ANONYMOUS, p. 562

AA Workshops, Roundups and Conventions serve many purposes and you'll never understand just how much you can get out of one of these events until you give a few of them a try. It doesn't have to cost you a lot of money or time either. Start with something local and work your way out from there. The types of events can run across a very wide spectrum, from a local workshop on the 4th Step or Getting into Service Work to the International Convention of Alcoholics Anonymous that takes place every 5 years in a different major city.

So, what's the point? Well, it's an opportunity to once again get further immersed in the Fellowship. You are outside of a structured meeting, at least part of the time, and have an opportunity to both meet new people in the program and further get to know people in the program that you may already have an acquaintance with. It's also an opportunity to broaden your knowledge and understanding of the program and how it works as nearly all of these Workshops, Roundups and Conventions have an educational element to them. Whether you are interested in learning more about the Traditions, the History of AA, Sponsorship, Service Work, or Spirituality - there is likely going to be something for you to grab a hold of there and many other like-minded people for you to meet and form bonds with.

So, how do you find out about these events? It's hard not to actually. Many of them are announced during or after meetings. There are also generally flyers lying around meeting rooms for upcoming conferences in the area that are recovery-related. Also, you can check your local Intergroup flyer, if they have one, or Intergroup Website. Finally, check other websites that list AA Conferences and Events (See Useful Resources Section for a nice list). I have been to many of these and, despite sometimes not wanting to go, enjoyed myself immensely once I was there. In fact, you may even want to consider volunteering to "work" if you have a great amount of anxiety about attending one of these events alone. This will get you in the door, keep you busy and provide you with instant introductions to others in the program. Most importantly, sign up, attend and get involved.

It is good to have an end to journey towards; but it is the journey that matters, in the end. -Ursula K. LeGuin

7 - Use the Telephone - Telephone Therapy 101

Almost without exception, alcoholics are tortured by loneliness Even before our drinking got bad and people began to cut us off, nearly all of us suffered the feeling that we didn't quite belong. AS BILL SEES IT, p. 90

If you've been to enough meetings, then you know about the telephone numbers. In a lot of meetings, when a newcomer raises their hand, a phone list will go around and people (same sex) will put their names and numbers on that list to give to that person afterwards so that they can call for support. Some meetings even have pre-printed phone lists of home group members that are ready for the taking. The tradition of "telephone therapy" goes back to the beginning of Alcoholics Anonymous, where Bill W. used the pay phone in the lobby of the Mayflower Hotel in Akron in 1935, looking for help when he felt like picking up a drink. This led to his first meeting with Dr. Bob, and eventually to the founding of AA. Dr. Bob, in later years, became one of AA's leading advocates of "telephone therapy".

So, why the phone numbers and insistence that we call others in the program? Well, there are several reasons. One is to gradually re-build your social circle with other people in recovery, including people who can act as a support system in time of need. The suggestion that we call others from the beginning is so that we get into the habit of doing this so that it is that much easier to do when there is a real need present. When you feel like picking up, it's much better if the last 10 people that you called in your phone are Program people and not old drinking buddies or your dealer.

Restart Your Recovery

I understand completely the awkwardness and uncomfortable feeling that comes with, first, asking someone else for their phone number and, second, actually calling them on the phone. Asking for phone numbers is very commonplace in AA and most people will give theirs out without a second thought. Also, calling someone else gets easier with practice as well and the conversations do not need to last a long time. You can simply say "Hi, this is ____ from the meeting and I'm just calling to check in. How are you doing?" That's just about good enough. The other person will generally take it from there and most people understand that many of us are uncomfortable with the phone.

So, if you are planning to Restart your recovery, one suggestion is to start using the telephone again. You can break out the phone list that you have crumpled in the drawer and start making use of it, ask some people before or after a meeting for their numbers or be extra bold and make an announcement when you share at a meeting. In the course of letting people know "where you're at" and what you're doing, just let the room know that you would really appreciate some phone numbers of people who would be willing to take calls. You'll likely either get a written list at the end of the meeting or be rushed afterwards. The most important part of this exercise, however, is to start using those numbers right away. Commit to call at least two people in the program, besides your sponsor, per day just to say "hi" and check in. You'll be amazed how much easier it gets and at where those simple phone calls will take you.

Taite Adams

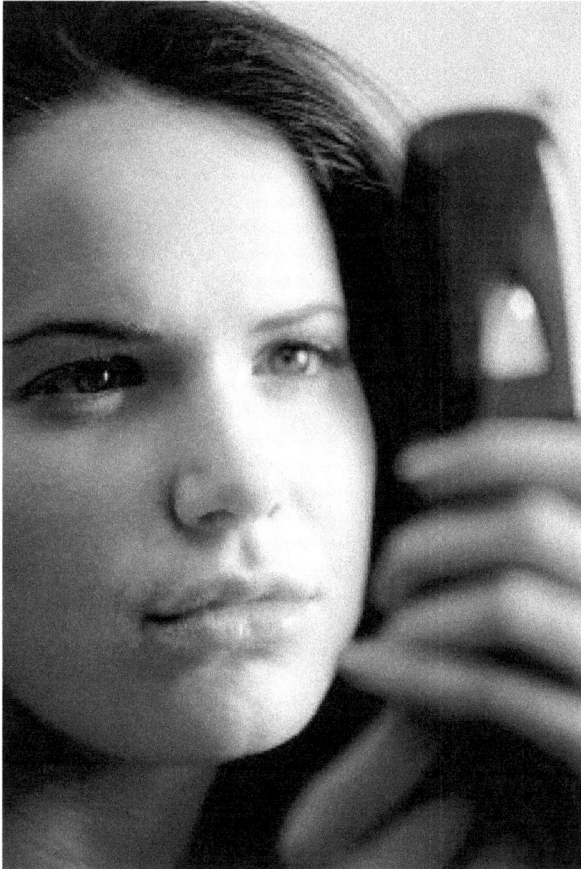

There are no problems we cannot solve together, and very few that we can solve by ourselves. -Lyndon B. Johnson

8 - Practice Prayer and Meditation

We're not cured of alcoholism. What we really have is a daily reprieve contingent on the maintenance of our spiritual condition. - Alcoholics Anonymous p. 85

The first thing that goes out the window as we move away from our recovery program and start down the road to relapse is Spirituality. We "take our will back", start running the show again, and profess that we've "got this". Well, as our emotional bottom has likely made it clear, or whatever else you'd like to label that kick in the teeth that made you realize you needed to make some changes, pretending to be in control wasn't working - again. Turning our back on spiritual principles leads to a virtual hornet's nest of unmanageability in nearly every area of living - career, finances, relationships, and just general peace of mind. This may be a point at which we begin to see, once again, that we are powerless over so much, and that again our lives have become unmanageable.

Should you need a reminder for expediency's sake, here it is: 12 Step programs, like AA, are not religious in nature at all. Rather, they are spiritual as members are able to form their own conception of a higher power as they see fit. The crux of the recovery program, once again, is the essence of learning to rely on a higher power and coming to realize that "I'm not it". Returning to AA, going to meetings, and Reworking the Steps will likely result in a return to prayer and meditation but I'd be remiss if I didn't give this the attention it deserves because "it's all spiritual" in the end, right?

Prayer and meditation have both been found to have great physical benefits as well as emotional and mental benefits. People who pray and meditate tend to be happier and are more resilient and resourceful in the face of problems. Clinical studies have shown that people who pray and meditate are more relaxed and have stronger immune systems, so they are less likely to be sick and are able recover from illnesses more easily if they do get sick. So, if we reap all of these benefits from it, why do we stop doing it? Again, it's a matter of priorities and instincts gone astray.

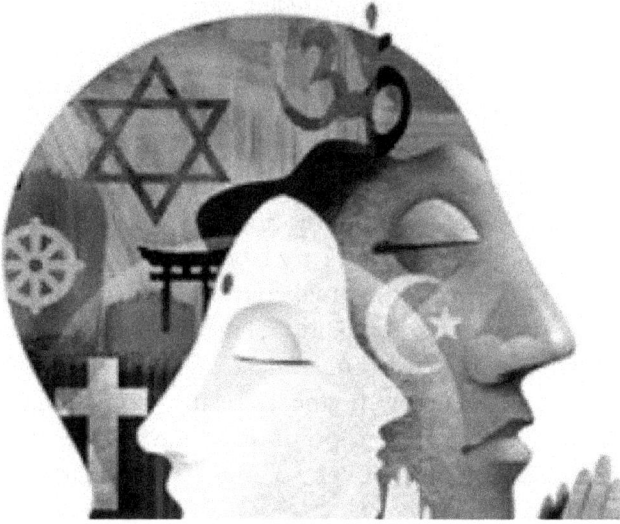

When I first got sober, I was told to get on my knees in the morning each day and ask God to keep me sober and then again at night and thank him for another day of sobriety. After a few years, I got a bit too busy for this as well. I can tell you that, today, this is something that I make time for each and every day and it is once again an essential part of my recovery program and my daily living. I remember being in control being a big issue for me when I got sober, in that it was a huge relief to finally admit that I wasn't in control and had no idea what was best for me. I call this "Practice Prayer and Meditation" so that I remember that it's a lifetime pursuit. It's nice to be able to get back to the feelings of peace of serenity that I once achieved through prayer and meditation and it takes only an ounce of willingness to make a start - again.

If God is your co-pilot, SWITCH SEATS!!!

Attend 12-Step Spiritual Retreats

Every now and again take a good look at something not made with hands - a mountain, a star, the turn of a stream. There will come to you wisdom and patience and solace and, above all, the assurance that you are not alone in the world. -Sidney Lovett

There is a quote that I love from the Language of The Heart -- *"How often do we sit in AA meetings and hear the speaker declare, 'But I haven't yet got the spiritual angle.' Prior to this statement, he had described a miracle of transformation which had occurred in him - not only his release from alcohol, but a complete change in his whole attitude toward life and the living of it. It is apparent to nearly everyone else present that he has received a great gift; 'except he doesn't seem to know it yet!'"* I can completely relate to this sort of statement because, despite all of the miracles that have occurred in my life since getting sober, I still question my spiritual progress and spiritual condition and try to find "things" that I can do to enrich it, which in itself may not always be a bad thing.

One activity I have found immensely helpful is attending 12 Step Spiritual Retreats. These can be short 1-day retreats to longer 3-day (long weekend) retreats or even week-long retreats in some places. These sorts of retreats provide many different experiences but they all offer both a "time out" from life's daily stresses as well as an opportunity to broaden and deepen one's own spiritual experience and understanding. There are different types of retreats available, some with workshops, some completely silent and others that offer spiritual counseling and meetings.

These retreats are great renewal tools and a fantastic way to meet new people in your area who are on the same spiritual journey. I have attended some at a Catholic Monastery and others at more wooded, camp-like settings. Check out the Useful Resources Section for links to find one near you or keep an eye out at your local meetings as they are often announced there as well.

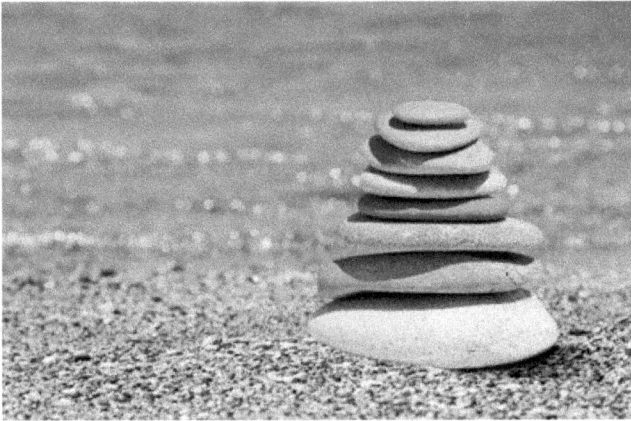

Other Meetings and Spiritual Pursuits

To keep the lamp burning we have to keep putting oil in it. -Mother Teresa

There are many "other" things that you can do in recovery to broaden your spiritual horizons and many people that are active in AA are also very active in other activities. Nothing precludes you from staying involved in your local church or from joining a church just because you are in recovery. In fact, many people in recovery are very active in their church. A popular church for recovering people in several places that I have lived is the Unity Church, probably because it is very inclusive and makes everyone feel welcome.

There are also other meetings that focus more on spiritual matters, some more bible-centric than others. **The Sermon on the Mount** is a popular meeting that studies the book by Emmet Fox. I have attended one of these meetings off and on for quite a few years and it has helped me tremendously with my views towards spirituality and my general outlook on life. Another meeting that you may be able to find locally is called **"A Course in Miracles"**, which is a study group of the book by Helen Schucman about finding spiritual transformation through forgiveness.

Meditation Meetings have also become very popular in many 12 Step rooms. These are meetings that are not necessarily AA meetings but are recovery-related guided meditation meetings. I have only been to a few of these but have enjoyed them. I have also used meditation tapes and even a pretty nifty meditation app for the iphone that provides different lengths of meditations.

These are just a few suggestions for other meetings that you can take part in to add to your pursuit of spiritual enlightenment. You can find links to more information on these in the Useful Resources section at the end of the book.

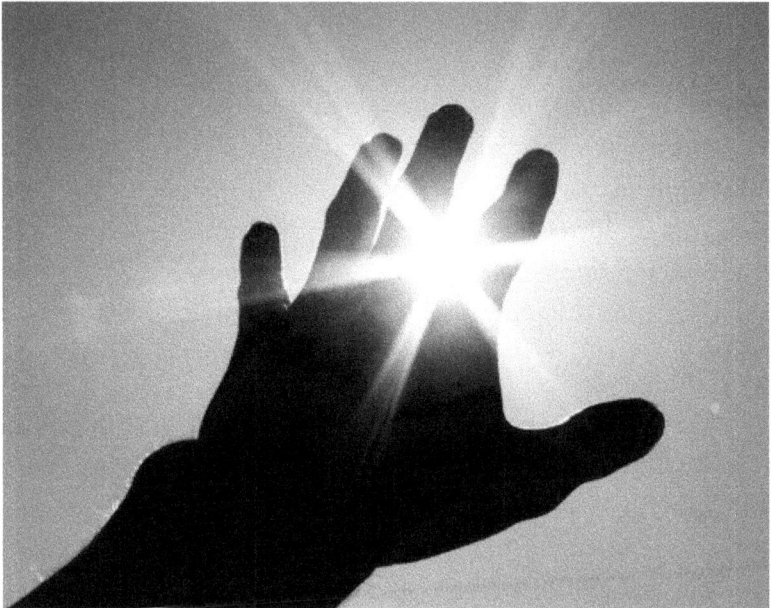

Practice Yoga

Try to be like the turtle - at ease in your own shell. *-Bill Copeland*

There is no doubt that yoga taps into mind, body and spirit and this is incredibly useful, and relevant, when we are talking about its practice with those in recovery from addiction. Unfortunately, a rather small percentage of those in 12 Step programs practice yoga, but this is changing. Yoga actually taps into the endocrine system and the nervous system and gets things moving in the right direction. It produces a euphoric effect and makes you feel great. Except with yoga, your body is left strengthened, your mind calm and your connection to everything, including your higher power, becomes clearer and sweeter.

Many of the ancient disciplines teach that true peace and happiness are only found within and cannot be achieved through outer means, such as turning outside of ourselves for substances. This makes them an excellent therapy for addiction recovery. The most profound teaching of many recovery therapies and yoga therapy is that a higher power exists within each and every one of us and sometimes it only needs nurturing to be awakened. Once awakened, it can guide one to a state of inner peace and freedom.

While going to your first Yoga class may sound scary, it's not that bad. Chances are you'll be able to find one of your buddies from a meeting who'd be willing to go with you or who already attends classes and would take you under their wing. I was dragged into my first class just this past year, and have to say that I was a bit skeptical. I actually thoroughly enjoyed the experience and have found Yoga to be both very peaceful and a nice challenge. I highly recommend it.

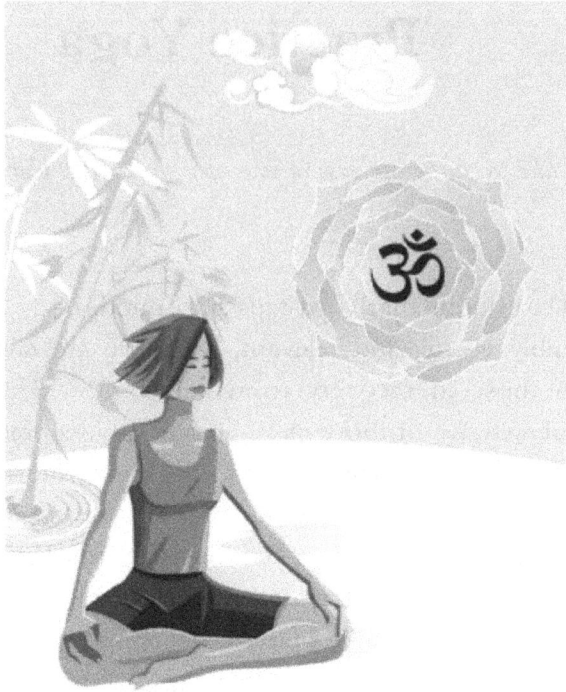

...the greater part of our happiness or misery depends on our dispositions and not on our circumstances. -Martha Washington

9 - Take Better Care of Yourself

The ultimate lesson all of us have to learn is unconditional love, which includes not only others but ourselves as well. -Elizabeth Kubler-Ross

When we first got sober, maybe in treatment or maybe with the guidance of a sponsor, we were probably given a crash course in basic "self care". This likely included basic instructions on how to do things like eat right, sleep right, wear clean clothes, and get a moderate amount of physical activity into your day. I can't speak for anyone else, but when sobriety lost its priority for me, some of these other things did too. My diet turned to crap, my sleep schedule was off and I stopped exercising altogether. My home and personal hygiene were passable but I'm not looking for snaps on those. I was pretty much a mess.

When I made the decision to do something different and restart my recovery and work on my emotional sobriety, I knew that there needed to be more involved than just the other things that we list in this book. I knew that I needed to start physically taking better care of myself. I was very overweight, tired all the time and had some physical problems that I know were not being helped by my diet. It was clear that just about anything would be a vast improvement over where I was at and so, one day, I just made that beginning. And it has made   all   the   difference.

Why Diet Matters

Better keep yourself clean and bright; you are the window through which you must see the world. -George Bernard Shaw

Many people in early recovery are told that they have a license to eat as much sugar as they want as it keeps the cravings at bay. This is only true to an extent and can actually set up some new, very unhealthy, eating habits in the recovering person.   In fact, a healthy diet with balanced nutrition helps improve mood and overall health in recovering people.   What's more important is to establish good eating habits and stick to them, just like the other healthy new habits that we pursue in recovery. Some general guidelines for diet are:

- Stick to regular mealtimes
- Eat a low-fat diet
- Get more protein, complex carbohydrates, and dietary fiber
- Vitamin and mineral supplements may be helpful during recovery (this may include B-complex, zinc, and vitamins A and C)

Regular meals for people in recovery are very important because we tend to get cranky, emotional and just plain confused when we are hungry.   Remember the acronym HALT (Hungry, Angry, Lonely, Tired)? That first one is important.   Other things to remember are to stay hydrated, eat healthy snacks and cut down on the caffeine.

When I decided to make changes in my diet, I didn't have to do a lot for there to be vast improvements. I was drinking too much caffeine and too much sugary soda. I was also eating absolutely no fruits or vegetables. I simply cut way back on the sodas, sugar and caffeine and added some greens to my diet. I didn't turn vegan (though I admire those that do), go on Weight Watchers or stop eating cheeseburgers. I didn't have to - or want to. Some small changes in diet and exercise made a huge difference in the way I looked and felt, both inside and out.

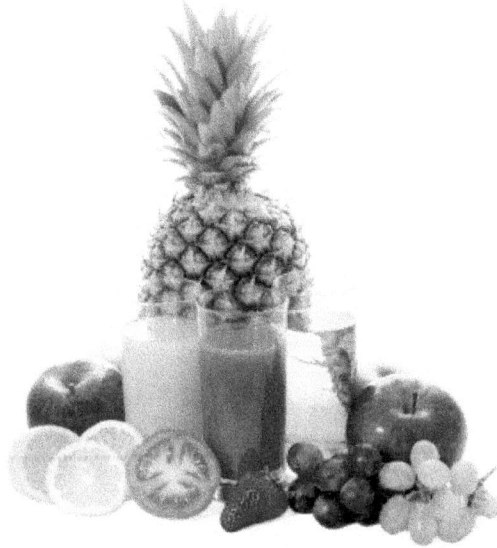

Exercise in Recovery

Self-discipline is self-caring. -M. Scott Peck

To say that I was out of shape when I began my journey back would be an understatement. I am honestly shocked that the muscles in my body didn't atrophy from disuse. I had literally spent several years at home in front of a computer for up to 15 hours a day, 6 days a week. There is no doubt in my mind that physical health and state of mind are vitally linked. When I am tired and don't feel well, my mind isn't as focused and I certainly have a much harder time seeing beauty and joy in the world. There is a definite emotional sobriety link here. So, that's my take on it, but what about the official word?

According to Dr. Nora Volkow of the National Institute on Drug Abuse, exercise can help relieve stress and reduce depression, both factors that can help reduce the rate of addiction. Exercise releases endorphins, which can elevate your mood and make you feel more confident in your recovery and help you to succeed. Dr. Volkow also notes that positive social interactions and staving off boredom are keys to successful addiction recovery. Exercise in a group setting, such as group runs or yoga, can provide a sober social setting, which improves the chance that recovery will be permanent.

Exercise works in a number of ways to help you feel better. Mark A. Smith, professor of neuroscience at Davidson University, notes that exercise actually mimics a lot of the same effects that drugs have on the brain, because exercise stimulates certain neurochemicals that sense pleasure. Exercise provides a "high" that could be important for addicts trying to combat cravings, experts say. In addition to decreasing anxiety and stress, physical activity helps increase levels of dopamine in the brain. Dopamine, a chemical that's associated with feelings of pleasure, is often diminished over time by substance abuse.

The different exercises that you do can have varied effects on your recovery. Cardio exercise can help you have more energy, burn fat and lose weight. Strength training exercises can help you develop muscle and increase your metabolism. You can try stretching exercises such as yoga and Pilates to quiet your mind and energize your body through sequential postures and breathing exercises.

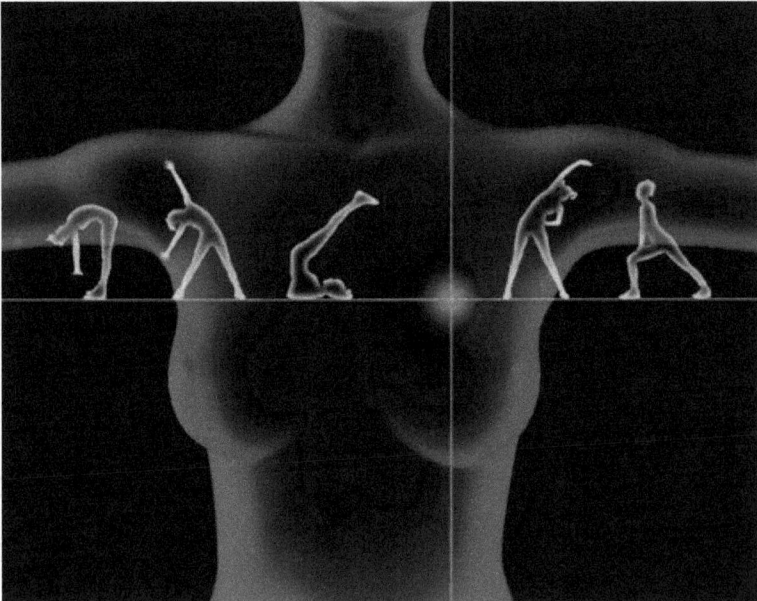

Some of these things may sound ominous but I made a very small start with this, which was all it took. I bought a small step machine for $40 or so at Walmart and began using it at home, able to only do 10-15 steps per day to start. I increased these by a few steps a day, until six months later I had a decent daily workout going and I decided to join a local gym. I felt so much better physically almost immediately and my confidence level and self-esteem went through the roof as people began to take notice of what I was doing and offer encouragement. While exercise by itself is no cure for addiction or emotional sobriety, it can be an additional tool to help build (or rebuild) a healthy life.

10 - A Change of Scenery

I have found that sitting in a place where you have never sat before can be inspiring. -Dodie Smith

Getting sober, and many times staying sober, is about forming new healthy habits and establishing a new consistency in life that emphasizes recovery and the fellowship of like-minded people. This does not mean, however, that we cannot have new experiences that can broaden our horizons and take us to new places. Quite the opposite. In fact, we're told that there is no place we cannot go and nothing that we won't be able to do should we have the right motives and be working to maintain our spiritual condition.

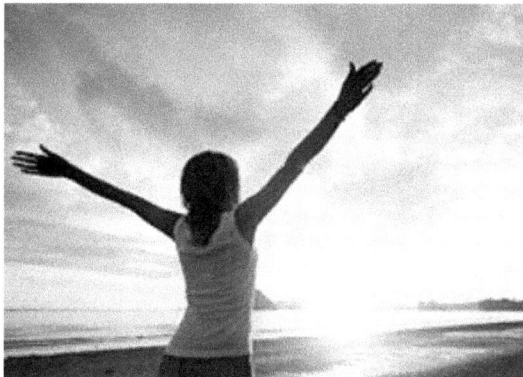

When I first got sober, I saw myself to be on very shaky ground and did not leave the safety of my county for the first year or do anything as daring as go out to a restaurant that served alcohol without other people in the program. As time went on, however, I became

more comfortable in my skin and was able to do many more things in sobriety, including travel and eventually move to a different area. While some of us may feel that we are, again, on shaky ground as we Restart our recovery, don't forget that we are able to do any of these things in sobriety with the right motives and can find them to be very enlightening, recharging and inspiring. However, before you pack your bags, be sure that you are making the right moves for your particular recovery and life situation.

Take a Sober Vacation

Life is either a daring adventure or nothing. -Helen Keller

Many of us dream of once again being able to go on vacations or, better yet, having the ability to take those trips that we only talked about while sitting on the barstool but were too bogged down with our addictions to take. Well, fear not - the sober travel business is HUGE. Choices abound as to what you can do with yourself stone cold sober these days and the sky is the limit. You can do whatever comes to the imagination, but there are things organized as diverse as sober music festivals, camping, yoga retreats and cruises, vacation rentals and resorts and much more.

Organized sober travel will generally happen through a sober travel agent (there are tons), who can research AA meetings in the location, be sure that tour operators are aware that participants are in recovery, and set up sober activities. Some sober travel agencies will allow for payment plans so that you can plan your trips with sober groups well in advance and do things such as go on ski trips, golfing, rafting, cruises and even Club Med vacations.

Aside from the organized sober travel groups, most major cruise lines will have "Friends of Bill" meetings on board for anyone who wants to attend. I have been on A LOT of cruises in recovery and it's a comfort just to know that those meetings are there, as some cruise ships are hot beds of alcohol consumption and debauchery. I have always loved to travel but many of my trips were a blur or ended up being insanely expensive because of the alcohol bill at the end. Getting to travel and see new places, and re-experience old places, sober has been a blessing.

Restart Your Recovery

Depending on your circumstances as you Restart your recovery, a sober vacation may be in order to recharge and reconnect. However, if you haven't done this before, consider an organized "recovery vacation" as they are more structured and will have meetings already set up for you. I went on a Sober Cruise after just a few years sober and it was a lot of fun. I met a lot of new people from all over the country. We had meetings on the ship, ate together, went on excursions together and stayed in touch after the trip. I've also traveled around the world, both with companions and alone, in sobriety and have enjoyed myself immensely. It takes a lot of pressure off of the itinerary when you are not worried about hunting down that next drink or drug and can just relax and enjoy the ride. This is one of the biggest benefits of sobriety to me. Interested in taking a sober vacation but don't know where to start? Check out the Useful Resources section for some links and ideas.

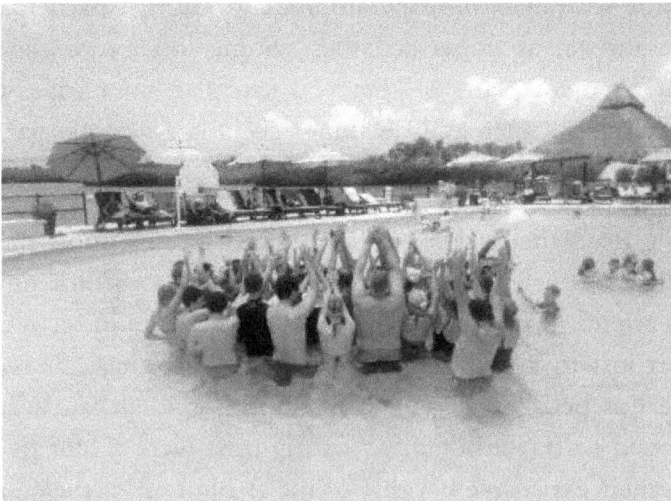

Permanent Change if Needed But Beware

"Sometimes you need to lose yourself, before you can find anything....."

I'm sure that I'm not the only person who tried a "geographic cure" while still drinking. Just a few years before I got sober, I became convinced that the city that I was living in was "the problem". I promptly quit my job, abandoned my home and moved to the other side of the state with my 2-year old child in tow, convinced that all of my troubles were in the rear-view mirror. Anyone who has heard the saying, "wherever you go, there you are", surely knows how that little exercise turned out. This is why I say "beware" when there is any suggestion of a permanent change of scenery.

However, sometimes in sobriety, we do move to a new area, start a new career or make a big change and this is just what the doctor ordered. The key here is to be doing these things for the right reasons and to not necessarily be convinced that the grass is going to be greener in someone else's pasture. The truth is that it won't be unless you are making changes from the inside out. It doesn't matter if the weather is nicer, if you have a better job, or are closer to your family - you will not be happier in a new place unless you are consistently taking action to further your spiritual development and growth. Also, don't forget that you can be just as isolated in your hometown as in someplace shiny and new.

So, why move at all then? Well, as we said, there are valid reasons for moving in recovery and people do it all the time. I moved at about 5 years sober but made the mistake of not putting any more effort into my program after I did. I didn't connect with people in the program or go to enough meetings so, when I decided to Restart my recovery, I had to start from scratch in this place that I had been living for quite some time. It was familiar surroundings but I really didn't know anyone or have any support system whatsoever. A new start can be accomplished anytime and in anyplace, whether you have just moved there or have been there for years.

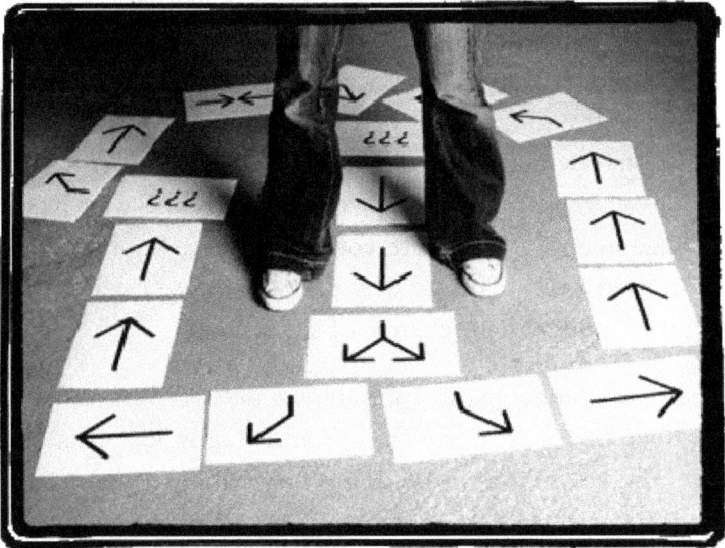

There is no such thing as a problem without a gift for you in its hands. -Richard Bach

11 - Write About It

All glory comes from daring to begin. -Eugene F. Ware

How many sponsors or therapists have recommended keeping a journal or "writing things down" to you? I know that I couldn't possibly count on two hands the number of times that I have been advised to put pen to paper and yet I still resist the exercise sometimes as being too bothersome. If I can write it down, surely I can just sit here on the couch and "think it" too, right? Well, there's a bit of a difference between the two and I do see this when lift my lazy hand and actually do the work.

We can self-reflect until we're blue in the face but the actual healing takes place when we are more easily able to organize our thoughts and emotions in a more coherent and manageable way. And the simple act of writing things down can accomplish this and provide a much-needed perspective. In fact, researchers have carried out a number of studies on journal writing and the role it can play in the restoration of good mental and physical health. What they have discovered is that keeping a written record of everything that is felt and experienced during recovery from a physical illness or a psychologically debilitating condition really does make a positive and lasting impact. Good physical and emotional health will empower any human being facing any type of daunting task or quest. As such, those tackling addiction issues are encouraged to make use of the spiritually transforming mind-body therapeutic effects of journal keeping.

Restart Your Recovery

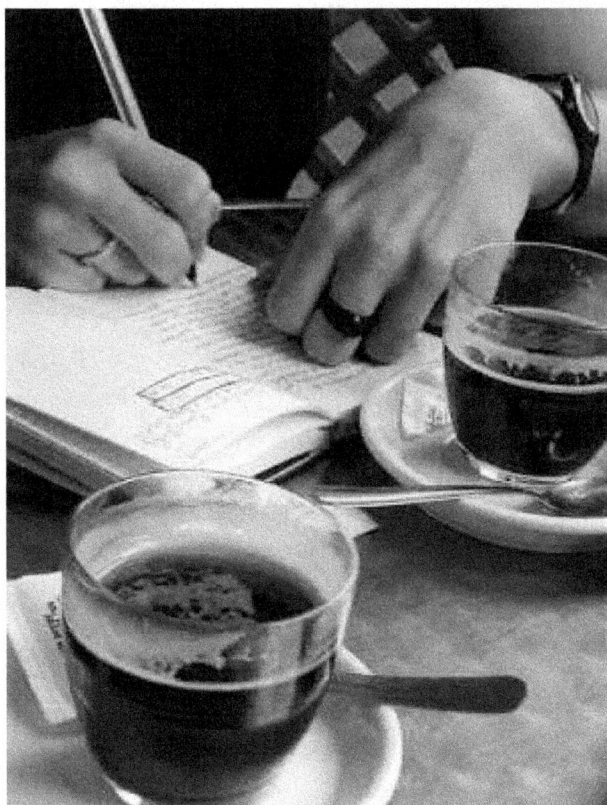

Keep a Recovery Journal

With the new day comes new strength and new thoughts. -Eleanor Roosevelt

Journal writing has proven to be such an important tool for addicts and alcoholics for several reasons. It allows us to analyze situations from either the past or present and to finally process those feelings. Think of the writing that we do when we are working the Steps. Journal writing can also help us to gain perspective, by allowing us to process feelings about things that have happened, or are happening, and then let them go. To many, a journal becomes something like a trusted friend, someone who will always give you the love and understanding that you desire as you struggle to make sense of your emotions and your circumstances. Here is a list of benefits of Journaling in Recovery:

- Keeping a journal means that people can learn more about themselves. When things are written down it makes it easier to observe patterns and find causes.
- Writing things down is a type of venting. Stress levels can be reduced because the individual is able to express their inner feelings externally. Just allowing emotions to pour out onto the paper can be very therapeutic.
- Keeping a journal increases accountability. By keeping a journal the individual is being more honest with themselves. They will be less able to use denial to ignore any bad behavior or unwise decisions.
- If people are feeling a lot of negativity it may be because they are misunderstanding the situation. By getting everything down on paper it makes things a lot clearer. This means that the individual will be less likely to act on their faulty interpretation of events.

- Writing down any goals in a journal increases the likelihood that they will be achieved. It may mean more successes and progress in recovery.

- Journaling is a wonderful way to track progress. It is nice to go back in time by reading older entries. The individual is able to see changes that they may not have otherwise noticed. People change slowly over time and it is easy to miss out on what has been achieved.

- This type of writing can be a way to come in closer contact with the subconscious. This can mean improved intuition and occasional life changing insights.

- Writing encourages people to think critically. Most people never examine their thoughts and assumptions. This means that they are usually functioning with a lot of flawed information influencing their decisions and actions.

- When the individual writes in their journal they have no need to worry about being judged. This can encourage them to be more open and honest with themselves.

- People in recovery can get periods where they are struggling to stay on course. By reading back on their journal entries they will be able to remind themselves of how far they have come. This can motivate them to re energize their efforts to build a life away from addiction.

So, as you are probably now sufficiently convinced to give this a shot, many people still don't know where to start. In fact, there is no wrong way to do this. There are many different forms of journaling that you can do, but some that may be of benefit to you include:

- **Stream of Consciousness Journal** - This is where you just sit down with your journal and pen and start writing whatever comes into your head. It's important not to make any edits to the writing and also not to worry about spelling, grammar or punctuation. (This is, in fact, the most common form of journaling and what I do when I write in my journal).

- **Diary Journal** - This is where people write down all of the important things that have happened each day. There can be a bit of "stream of consciousness" to this as well.
- **Gratitude Journal** - This is useful for people who suffer from a lot of negative thoughts and emotions, as it puts emphasis on the positive things in life (see next section of book).
- **Spiritual Journal** - This is where people write their observations on their spiritual development and activities related to their journey.
- **Exercise/Health Journal** - This type of journal outlines a person's efforts to live a healthy lifestyle.

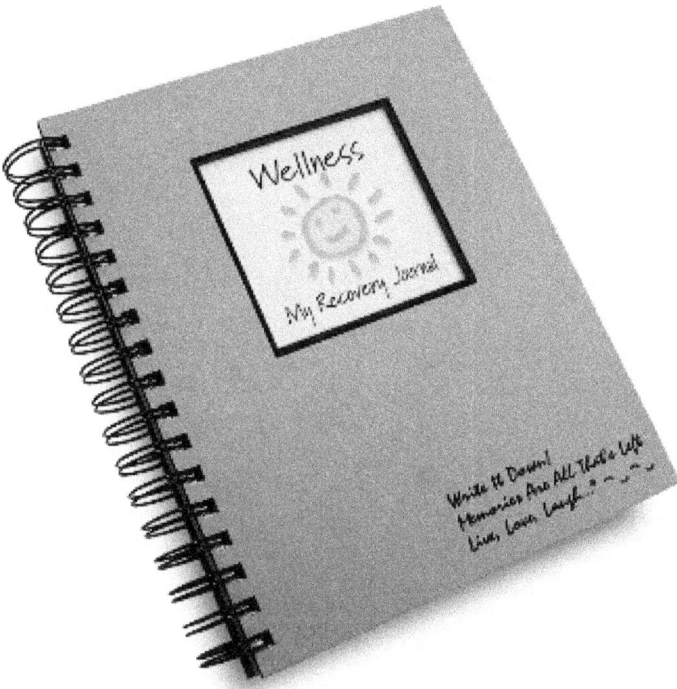

Your particular journal can be any of these, all of these, none of these, or any combination thereof. It's your tool to use in recovery and, for many of us, something new to help chart a new path and a fresh way of doing things. I have started and stopped journaling at different points in my sobriety but did begin doing this again regularly as I made a new beginning in recovery and it has been a very useful tool. Journal writing is a tool for empowerment, and if you are an addict it is a powerful method for coping and change that can help you overcome the deep pain and feelings of helplessness that have ruled your existence for far too long.

It is astonishing in this world how things don't turn out at all the way you expect them to! -Agatha Christie

Make Gratitude Lists

We can only be said to be alive in those moments when our hearts are conscious of our treasures. - Thornton Wilder

I remember when I first started coming to AA and heard people declare that they were "grateful recovering alcoholics". This baffled me. Not to mention the fact that my sobriety date is at the beginning of Gratitude Month - I really thought these people had gone off the deep end and that I was doomed to a life with a bunch of cream puffs. It didn't take much time for me to start changing my tune and to see that these people perhaps had gotten a hold of some pretty decent ideas - one of which being that "a full and thankful heart cannot entertain great conceits", which meant to me that I could find happiness and stay away from a drink if I could find enough to be grateful for. This generally wasn't always that difficult but, once again, often required me putting pen to paper.

Gratitude itself is defined as a feeling of thankfulness for a benefit that an individual has received. This can be interpreted many ways and very broadly - lucky for us. The purpose of the Gratitude List is to help the person recognize and focus on the good things that are in their life. As human beings, we have a tendency to take things for granted, and as addicts and alcoholics we can simply not see the forest for the trees at times. Keeping a record of things that we feel grateful for will ensure a continuing positive outlook on life. Here are some of the real benefits of keeping a Gratitude List:

- It is easy for people to begin taking their recovery for granted. A gratitude list will prevent this from happening.

- It is highly beneficial for people to keep a positive attitude in their recovery. Those who regularly think about the good things in their life will be able to maintain a positive attitude.
- Somebody is less likely to relapse if they are grateful for what they currently have.
- If the individual is having thoughts of relapse they will be able to read their gratitude list and be reminded of what they have to lose.
- It is easy for people to miss all the things they have to feel good about. A gratitude list will be a good reminder.
- This type of journaling can also be a good way for the individual to gauge their progress in recovery.

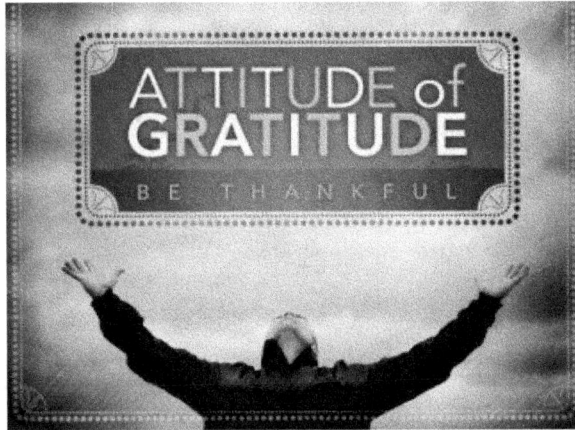

So, now that you are possibly convinced that this is a good idea (if not, ask your sponsor), just how do you go about making a Gratitude List? This doesn't have to be a daunting task and there are no hard and fast rules about it. However, here are some ideas that may get you started:

- The usual way to create a gratitude list is to just write down things in list form. This way the individual might only use one or two words to describe each thing they are grateful for.
- It is also possible for people to write a gratitude list in a longer form. Here they can describe in more detail each of the things they feel grateful about.
- In order for it to be effective the gratitude list is not something that people do once and then forget about. It should be updated regularly – at least once a week but many people will try to add to this list daily.
- It is a good idea to buy a nice notebook for these gratitude notes. It is likely going to be something that the individual will want to cherish.
- If people are having thoughts of drinking or using drugs again they should read back on their gratitude lists as parts of their relapse prevention plan.
- Modern technology means that there are now many options for people who want to create an electronic gratitude list.
- If people are unsure about what they should feel grateful about they will find plenty of examples of gratitude lists online.

A few additional notes on Gratitude Lists for the non-conventional folks out there:

- Something that I have heard in meetings several times that I found novel: Make a Gratitude List using the alphabet, finding something to be grateful for that starts with each letter of the alphabet as you go.
- If you can't find anything to be grateful for, make a list of the things that you are currently taking for granted. You'll find that the two lists are remarkably similar.

- My sponsor has me text her one thing that I am grateful for every single morning. She, in turn, texts me something that she is grateful for back. I have started using this tool with my sponsees and it's a great daily gratitude reminder.

This can be as simple or as complicated and elaborate as you wish to make it. You can incorporate your Gratitude List into your regular Recovery Journal or have a separate journal for it. You can simply pull out a scrap of paper and start writing. Remember, this isn't something that you do one time and are done with it. Alcoholics have short memories and we'll either need to refer back to the list often or simply re-write it when needed. Regardless, it's become clear over the years that there is ALWAYS something to be grateful for no matter what I may be going through and, should I simply be willing to sit down and go through this exercise, I'll realize that my life is really overflowing with blessings.

Gratitude unlocks the fullness of life. It turns what we have into enough, and more. It turns denial into acceptance, chaos to order, confusion to clarity. It can turn a meal into a feast, a house into a home, a stranger into a friend. -Melody Beattie

12 - Consider Outside Help

When you're drowning, you don't say 'I would be incredibly pleased if someone would have the foresight to notice me drowning and come and help me,' you just scream. -John Lennon

There is a lot of confusion and debate in recovery when it comes to "outside" issues and whether or not it is ok to ask for and pursue outside help and other things like medication.   I honestly can't picture anyone, myself included, who walked into AA or a treatment center with the only "problem" being that they had drank too much.   There are always underlying causes and conditions that got us to a particular point in time (hopefully a "bottom") and some of us used many different things to excess - alcohol, drugs, food, people.   Others of us may have additional psychiatric diagnoses that contributed to our disease and may also play a role in our recovery process and our emotional sobriety.   All of these are valid things to take a good hard look at and, if you go to a treatment center, they will certainly help you with this.   However, if you do not, you may be left even more lost and confused as to what to about these "other issues" as you move forward and make a new beginning in recovery.

It would be a product of false pride to claim that A. A. is a cure-all, even for alcoholism   AS BILL SEES IT, p. 285

Restart Your Recovery

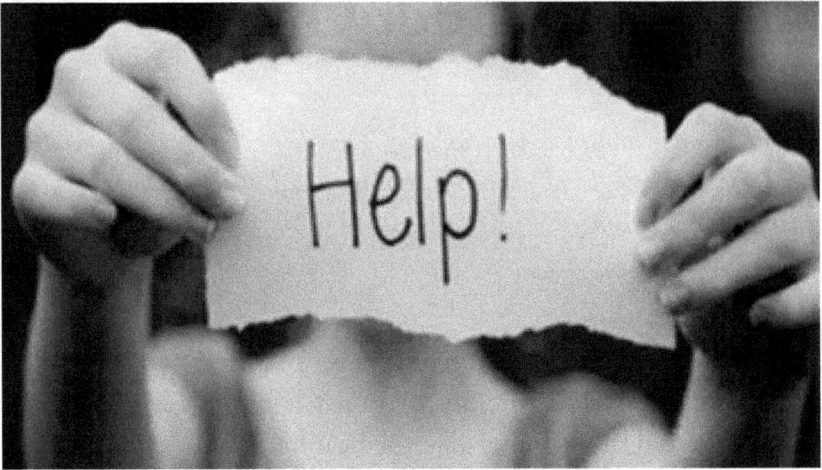

Go to Treatment (Again or For the First Time)

You are not responsible for your disease, but you are responsible for your behavior and consequently your recovery.

Many people who haven't picked up a drink or a drug wouldn't consider going to treatment - either again for the first time. However, there are people in the rooms (I know some) who profess a longing to "take a break" from society and the prospect of spending a few months away at a place like Cliffside Malibu sounds pretty alluring. Many people also never went to treatment before getting sober and feel like they "missed something". Perhaps they did - I passed through the doors of many treatment centers so feel like I've seen my fair share.

The truth of the matter is that it's certainly not going to cost you your sobriety if you do decide to check yourself into treatment to avoid relapse. It will, however, cost you a bit of time and money. Any experience is going to return dividends should you be willing to put in the effort and making it through a stay in even the nicest treatment center certainly requires a bit of effort. This is because they are all designed to take you out of your comfort zone, provide structure and make you take a good hard look at yourself. Could you do this at home? Yes, to an extent but probably not in this "boot camp", condensed, sort of format.

So why consider doing this at all if you are simply trying to Restart Your Recovery? Well, take a few minutes and consider just how far down that road to relapse scale you have gone and how close to picking up a drink or a drug you think you may be. Be really honest about this and consider pulling in some trusted friends, and your sponsor, for this discussion. Heck, stage your own mini-intervention if you must. If you see picking up a drink as "an inevitability", perhaps going to rehab to head that off may be a good idea. Remember, this is a deadly disease and we are supremely lucky to get another chance at life. There's no telling what can happen, who can be injured, or may die, once the line has been crossed. Be very honest in your self-appraisal and do what is right for your recovery.

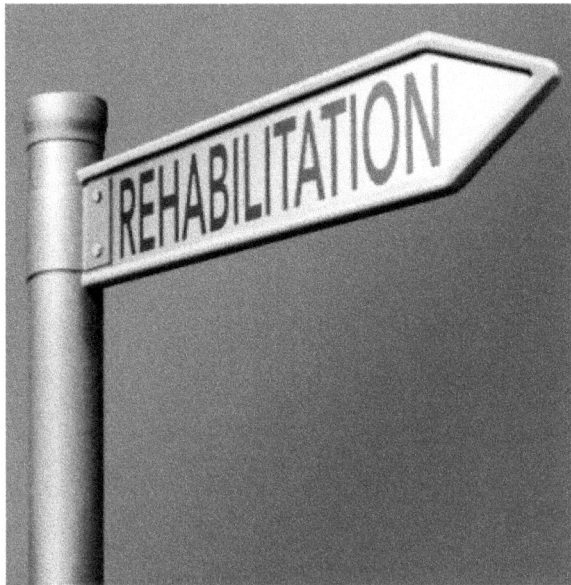

If you're going through hell, keep going. -Winston Churchill

Other Professional Help

Asking for help does not mean that we are weak or incompetent. It usually indicates an advanced level of honesty and intelligence. -Jim Rohn

Many people in recovery struggle in dealing what we call "outside issues". Some of these, such as other addictive behaviors, can be dealt with by working the Steps or through participation in another fellowship. Still others cannot and this is where confusion often sets in. The other issues that may be affecting a person's recovery and emotional sobriety may have been known in advance, may not come to light until well into sobriety, or may have been neglected for a time as a person stopped taking care of themselves or working their program. The fact is that addicts can be pretty complicated folks, and despite AAs success in helping alcoholics get and stay sober, AA alone is not enough to manage the host of complications that an alcoholic may have. That is why AA is very clear about separating itself from medicine and psychiatry, pointedly telling members to get "outside help" when necessary.

Research has proven that people with alcohol or other drug disorders often suffer from a bouquet of descriptive acronyms and psycho jargon that has replaced AAs placid "character defects" mentioned so often in the Big Book - "duel disorders," "comorbid disorders," "MICA" (mentally ill chemical abusers) and substance abusers with "SMI" (serious mental health illness), to name a few. The newest term is "co-occurring disorder." The percentages are a bit daunting as well; about 16% of the US population suffers from substance abuse problems. In people with mental health disorders, the number is almost twice as high: 29%. Forty-seven percent of schizophrenics and 56% of people with bipolar disorders have a substance abuse disorder. Almost 80% of alcoholics experience depression at some time in their lives, and 30% meet the diagnostic requirements for major depression. As many as one-third of people entering treatment for substance abuse issues meet the requirements for Post-Traumatic Stress Syndrome (PTSD).

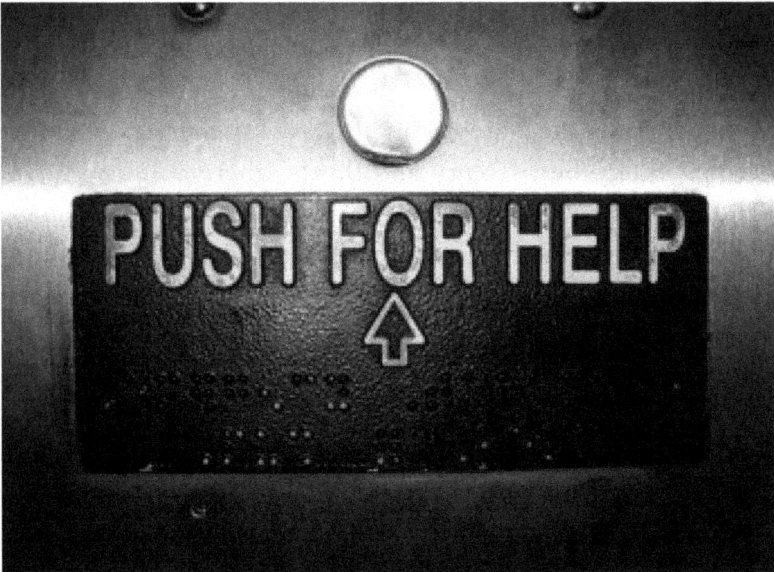

So how does a member know when it is time to seek "outside help"? Well, if you have been handed one of those nifty diagnoses either before getting sober, in treatment, or sometime since that would be a good indication that you may want to check in with your doctor and let them know what's up. If you don't have a specialist, just start with a General Practitioner and be honest about your situation and where you are at. A great mental health professional for recovering addicts are LADC's (Licensed Alcohol and Drug Counselor), which many times can either be psychiatrists or medical doctors with additional training in chemical dependency and abuse issues. It's well-known that diagnosing and treating many "co-concurring" disorders can be difficult until the patient has been sober at least 6 months, when you can get a clearer picture of what they are really like.

One of the many dangers of not managing co-occurring disorders, of course, is relapse. Active addiction amplifies the co-occurring disorders so that sobriety must indeed come first if the sufferer is going to have any hope of getting better. But the other side is that untreated depression, anxiety or mania can trigger relapse. The American Association of Marriage and Family Therapists has set up an online service for people in recovery to "seek outside help." The TherapistLocator.net website is designed specifically to put those in need of services in touch with those who provide them. If you feel like you need Outside Help, don't be afraid to get it.

Happiness is not something you postpone for the future; it is something you design for the present. -Jim Rohn

It All Comes Down to Willingness and Action

We must be content to grow slowly. Most of us will still barely be at the beginning of our recovery by the time we die. But that is better than killing ourselves pretending to be healthy. - Simon Tugwell

There are many many things that you can do to get back on the beam and Restart your journey in recovery. Do you need to do all of the things that are listed in this book? Probably not but it's suggested that you give some honest thought to each one of them and consider your reasons for not being willing to give them a try. Because it really all comes down to willingness and action. For most of us, something has occurred, or failed to occur, that has brought about enough pain for us to want to make a change. Should we call this an "emotional bottom"? Perhaps.

The truth of the matter is that we may still have a grip (barely) on physical sobriety but what we refer to as emotional sobriety has probably flown out the window long ago. This is the ability to be able to regulate our emotions and mood, to deal with strong feelings without resorting to compulsive or destructive behaviors. At this point, it may be just sleeping all the time or over-eating but that is likely just the tip of the iceberg should something not be done, and soon. I hate to use the word "dry drunk" but, hey - if it walks like a duck.

Maintaining emotional sobriety, and then spiritual growth, is a lifelong project and requires daily action. The actions that are required (or "suggested" if you prefer) are laid out in black and white and in list form in this very book. Some of the actions are meant to be distractive in nature, in that they take your mind off of your troubles, yourself, etc. Other actions are meant as a mechanism to rebuild the way we look at the world, ourselves and each other. The key element in both of these, however, is ACTION. You will get no relief and make no progress whatsoever if you are not taking action. It's that simple. It doesn't matter where you are at today, that is simply where you begin as you get this amazing chance to Restart Your Recovery.

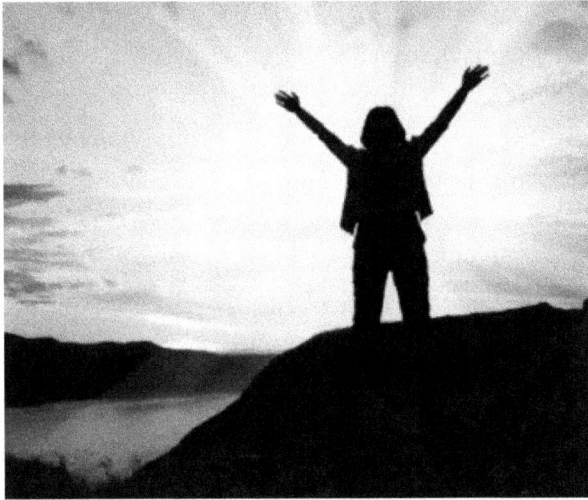

Real hope combined with real action has always pulled me through difficult times. Real hope combined with doing nothing has never pulled me through. - Jenni Schaefer

Useful Resources

Treatment Centers

There are no "public" websites that offer treatment center, detox and sober living directories. Unfortunately, any site you find will be filled with "sponsored results". This means rehabs that have paid for ad space. That's not always a bad thing, just not an unbiased thing. The best site I've found is Sober.com. You'll get the sponsored results in your search but you will also get all of the public listings as well, including the government-funded (some free) facilities.

Another Treatment Center Resource (http://www.drugrehabcenters.org/ByState/Drug_Rehab_Centers_With_Sliding_Scale_Fees.htm) - This one also lists the treatment centers that either have a sliding fee scale, accept public funds or are free.

Support Groups

Alcoholics Anonymous (aa.org)
Al-Anon Websites (al-anon.alateen.org)
Narcotics Anonymous (na.org)
Cocaine Anonymous (ca.org)
Adult Children of Alcoholics (adultchildren.org)
Co-Dependence Anonymous (CoDA) (coda.org)

Workshops, Roundups and Conventions

AA Grapevine Calendar of Events (aagrapevine.org/calendar)
AA Events around the world

United States Recovery (usrecovery.info/Events)
Recovery Related Events (Various Fellowships - Mostly U.S. and Canada)

Step12.com (step12.com/aa-conventions)
AA Conventions, Conferences and Round-ups, including Big Book and 4th Step Workshops

Alcoholics Anonymous Europe Events (aa-europe.net)

Retreats and Yoga

Retreat Finder (retreatfinder.com)
This is the most comprehensive world-wide listing of retreats that you will find anywhere, with literally thousands to chose from. Be aware, however, that these are not all 12-Step retreats so do your research on them as you search.

The following are more recovery-focused retreats:

Wisconsin Agape (wisconsinagape.org)
Located in a wooded rural setting near Milwaukee, weekend 12 step retreats for members of all recovery fellowships are held four times a year. Long format marathon meetings allow for in depth sharing. The suggested donation for the weekend is $50.

12 Step Retreats (12stepretreat.org)
Located in the Santa Cruz mountains of northern California, the retreat is held on 67 mountain acres at the Presentation Retreat & Conference Center. Experienced retreat leaders guide participants through the principles and steps of the 12-step program in five one-hour talks. There are scheduled meetings for AA, Al-Anon, and sharing meetings, with additional rooms available for NA, Nar-Anon and other 12 step meetings.

Casa   Hamaca
Guesthouse (casahamaca.com/Pages/Offer.Sober.html)
Casa Hamaca in the Yucatan of Mexico is geared toward sober travel.
In May, 2010 they held their first sober retreat called Recovery &
Discovery Retreat Week, designed as a physical, mental, emotional and
spiritual experience to facilitate meaning in one's daily life. The retreat
includes fellowship, meetings, twelve step work and climbing pyramids.
Quarterly retreats are planned.

Dan Anderson Renewal Center at
Hazelden (hazelden.org/web/go/renewalcenter)
Situated on Hazelden's 500-acre wooded campus in Center City, MN,
the Renewal Center provides a peaceful setting for group interaction or
private times of reflection. Retreat structures are flexible and can
include one of their special Recovery Retreat programs or day, week or
longer stays as part of one's ongoing recovery program. These retreats
are designed to meet the spiritual recovery needs of individuals who are
actively involved in any Twelve-Step program. Guests do not have to
be Hazelden alumni to participate.

Jesuit Retreat House (jesuitretreathouse.org/retreats.cfm)
This Catholic retreat house located in Oshkosh, Wisconsin welcomes
people of all faiths to their four-day and eight-day retreats. Specific
retreats are designated for men and women in 12-Step recovery
programs.

New Beginning Ministry (newbeginningmin.org)
Located in Wayne County, PA, this retreat program is a faith-based
twelve-step program for recovery. It offers a safe and structured
environment for those with substance addiction to learn about the
problem of addiction, the solution to addiction, and the program of
action that leads to change. Recovery retreats are in a residential
community for alcohol and drug dependence. New Beginning
represents a non-medical approach to alcohol and drug addiction based
on a spirit-centered community.

Open Door Retreat (opendoorretreat.com)
Run by a certified alcohol and drug counselor and certified equine
therapist, this program for women in recovery offers week-long
retreats in a peaceful setting in Mexico. Retreats are scheduled twice a

month. The weekly rate is $1,900 double occupancy. The retreat focuses on a holistic approach to recovery and personal growth including meditation and relaxation, 12 step meetings, massage, yoga, the arts, cooking classes and other supportive activities.

Retreats Online (retreatsonline.com)
Covers a wide variety of retreat experiences including spiritual/religious retreats, nature retreats, health and wellness retreats and others in the U.S., Canada, Asia, Europe and the UK.

Serenity Retreat League (serenityretreatleague.org)
Founded by the late Father Frederick G. Lawrence in 1964 at the request of an Al-Anon group, Serenity Retreats now serve members of many Twelve Step programs. These retreats are an extension of the spiritual growth nurtured by all Twelve Step fellowships and pursued by each individual in his or her own way. Serenity Retreats are nondenominational, ecumenical and spiritual rather than specifically religious. The leaders may be Catholic, Protestant, Jewish ministers or laypersons. Only spiritual leaders familiar with Twelve Step programs lead Serenity Retreats. Click on Scheduled Retreats in the left menu bar for an online list of retreats organized by month or by location.

Total   Health   Recovery
Program (totalhealthrecoveryprogram.com)
This holistic recovery program integrates spirituality, addiction and holistic treatment to provide the opportunity for profound healing. THRP offers a two week residential substance abuse program which is held at Sunrise Springs, a retreat center. Diagnostic, assessment and treatment protocols consist of live cell blood analysis, saliva and neurotransmitter assessments, massage, acupuncture, chiropractic, yoga, and meditation, among other approaches. Programs are held when enough people sign up for a recovery program.

Transformations   Spirituality   Center,   Sisters   of   St.
Joseph (transformationscenter.org/12step-2.htm)
Located in southwest Michigan, this interfaith spiritual community offers retreats for men and women in recovery from alcohol addiction. The focus is to help those in recovery discover new levels of the 12

step philosophy in a quiet atmosphere led by experienced 12 step facilitators. There are evening long mini-retreats as well as full day and weekend retreats, all focusing on specific areas of recovery.

Serenity Retreats (serenityretreats.eu)

Located in the picturesque southwest of Ireland on the Maharees peninsula, Serenity Retreats is a family-run support service with over 20 years of personal and professional experience with addiction issues. All retreats offer workshops, daily recovery meetings and guided meditations on the beach. Perfect for individuals, couples, and small groups, the hotel accommodates up to 16 people at a time.

Wisconsin Agape (wisconsinagape.org)

Located in a wooded rural setting near Milwaukee, weekend 12 step retreats for members of all recovery fellowships are held four times a year. Long format marathon meetings allow for in depth sharing. The suggested donation for the weekend is $50.

Sober Holidays (soberholidays.ie)

Sober Holidays provides alcohol free holidays in the hills of Monchique close to the coast on the Algarve in Portugal. This holiday/retreat is suitable for people in recovery from addiction or anyone who cannot or does not want to drink alcohol. Sober holidays and sober retreats are important for people in the early stages of recovery from addiction and/or illness.

Yoga Farm Retreats (sivananda.org/farm)

Located in the Sierra foothills of Northern California, the Yoga, Ayurveda and 12 Step Recovery Retreat is offered two times a year. The retreat is based on the 4 Paths of Yoga, 5 Points of Yoga, Ayurveda, Svastha (being established in the self) and Meditation. The therapists are active members of 12 step programs and the retreat offers an opportunity to relate 12 step work to the ancient teachings of yoga and Ayurveda in order to provide a strong foundation for wellness and a deepening spiritual practice. Their other ashrams in the Bahamas, New York and Canada may also be offering this retreat in the future.

Yoga

Yoga Of Recovery (yogaofrecovery.com)
Yoga of Recovery is a retreat integrating the wisdom of Yoga and Ayurveda (the traditional medicine of India) with the tools of 12-Step Recovery. Yoga postures and breathing help strengthen the physical body for those healing from addiction. Ayurveda works at healing and purifying the body and mind through practical advice on diet and lifestyle. The retreat also offers daily 12-Step meetings focused on experience, strength and hope, vegetarian meals, and other tools of recovery including meditation training and positive thinking. Retreats are offered throughout the U.S. and internationally. A schedule is available online.

Tommy Rosen's Recovery 2.0 (tommyrosen.com)
Recovery 2.0 is all about sharing the gifts of yoga and meditation with people in recovery from addictions and with others who desire to get past any hurdle that stands between them and their happiness.

Other Meetings and Spiritual Resources

Sermon on the Mount (emmetfoxmeetings.com)

If you are interested in learning more about the spiritual teachings of Emmet Fox, check out this great new website dedicated to bringing people together for just that purpose. They have a Facebook Page as well.

A Course in Miracles (acim.org)

As its title implies, the Course is arranged throughout as a teaching device. It consists of three books: a 622-page Text, a 478-page Workbook for Students, and an 88-page Manual for Teachers. The order in which students choose to use the books, and the ways in which they study them, depend on their particular needs and preferences. Although Christian in statement, the Course deals with universal spiritual themes. It emphasizes that it is but one version of the universal curriculum. There are many others, this one differing from them only in form. They all lead to God in the end.

Unity Church (unity.org)

Unity is a center of spiritual light for people of the world. We are dedicated to letting this light shine so brightly that people become more aware of their spiritual nature and express it in their daily lives. We address physical, mental and emotional needs through affirmative prayer and spiritual education. We serve those who seek inspiration and prayer support as well as those who use Unity teachings as their primary path of spiritual growth.

Sober Travel Resources

Travel Agencies

In This Life Custom Getaways: (inthislife.com)

The staff of In This Life handle all types of travel arrangements — including cruises, safaris, and custom getaways. Their primary focus is to create and organize trips for people in 12-step recovery programs but they also help plan international tours and local sailing expeditions for singles, couples, and bigger groups. Clients have been enjoying their annual Sober Safaris— where a group of travelers in recovery heads to Kenya for breathtaking views of Mt. Kilimanjaro and eye-opening trips into the Amboseli and Aberdare National Parks— for years. Other trips, planned specifically for sober people but with other folks on board, include getaways to Greece, Spain, and more.

California Sober Travel: (californiasobertravel.com)

California Sober Travel isn't just for Californians but for anyone interested in living the sober lifestyle and traveling with like-minded people. Two of their most popular trips are sober cruises along the Mexican Riviera and vacation rentals at locations around the world (Maui, Florida, or the Mayan Riviera). A great way to make new friends, Sober Travel offers group travel in all sizes. They also arrange meetings and guest speakers on all of their trips (group leaders are all AA members).

<u>Sober Vacations International</u>: (sobervacations.com)

Sober Vacations work to expand travelers' comfort zones while incorporating recovery into every trip. Sober Club Med — where travelers head to the famous Club Med in Turks & Caicos for an all-sober week filled with meetings, meditation groups, and nightly entertainment — was their first vacation and remains their most popular trip. They also have rafting excursions to the Grand Canyon, golfing weekends in Utah, and Alaskan cruises.

Resorts and Hotels:

<u>The Aerie Inn of Vermont</u>: (aerieinnofvermont.com)

This charming inn that was a frequent vacation spot for Bill W. and Lois when they were alive offers activities on the water at Emerald Lake as well as hiking in the nearby Green Mountains. Guests can also explore the history of East Dorset—home of the Vermont Summer Festival. Even better for AA history nuts: travelers can visit the birthplace of Bill W. and even attend AA or Al-anon meetings at the Wilson House. Accommodating both sober and non-sober guests, The Aerie has space for up to 36 people (camping options are also available).

<u>Cortijo El Saltador</u>: (elsaltador.com)

An Andaluz farmhouse situated in a silent valley between the desert of Tabernas and the beaches of Cabo de Gata in Spain, this hotel offers healthy Mediterranean foods, special diets, homeopathic detox programs and a lot of individual space in a friendly, safe environment. They also have massage and osteopath treatments (an alternative form of manual medicine where the body is taught how to heal itself), yoga classes, and guided hikes and climbing. The house fits up to 20 people, and though there is nothing specifically offered on the

12-steps, it's often rented by sober groups looking for a beautiful and meditative retreat in one of the world's most stunning locations.

Fourth Dimension Resort: (fourthdimensionresort.com)

This eight-person resort in Tamarindo, Costa Rica has a mission: to provide a safe and comfortable place for adults seeking a vacation in a tropical climate that includes adventures, activities and fellowship in a sober and serene environment. Located on the northwest coast of Costa Rica in Central America, the Fourth Dimension Resort requests that its guests remain drug and alcohol free for their stay in the lodge. It's privately secluded on 28 acres of serene forest, but is only 15 minutes from town — which is filled with beaches, restaurants, shops and beautiful sunsets.

Sober Haven Bali: (soberhavenbali.com)

A boutique hotel on the Indonesian island of Bali created especially for travelers participating in 12-step programs and dedicated to sober living, Sober Haven provides an enchanting space for sober folks to surf, scuba dive, tour, and golf. The resort also offers yoga, delicious meals, and decadent spa treatments. Short stays and longer retreats are both possible.

Rancho de Caldera (ranchodecaldera.com)

An environmentally friendly boutique resort catering to those who want an extraordinary, healthy and sober getaway. Located in the mountains of western Panama.

Cruises:

Sober Cruises: (sobercruises.com)

The Sober Cruises committee is an organizer of Round Ups, organized 12-step convention-like events, for people in recovery programs, AA, Al-Anon, and their friends and family members. Each Round Up has been structured and crafted "for, by, and about" 12-step programs and its members. Though the cruises do include non-sober folks not affiliated with any 12-step or sober programs, these Round Ups on the water maintain a commitment to sober living and principles while traveling the globe. Trips include cruises to the Caribbean, Canada, Alaska, and Catalina Island.

Sober Celebrations: (sobercelebrations.com)

Looking for less meetings, more shuffleboard? Sober Celebrations is all about the fun. Groups can range from more intimate gatherings of friends to larger expeditions that provide new opportunities for fellowship amongst strangers. All cruises are on conventional cruise lines, which do include non-sober passengers. But with cruises to the Mediterranean, up the Viking River, and through the Alaskan glaciers, who needs a drink?

Adventure Tourism:

Easy Does It Adventures: (easydoesitadventures.com)

Easy Does It Adventures, LLC creates unique group travel vacations for 10-20 folks at a time, providing an ideal opportunity to meet new sober friends who also want to indulge their wild side. Possibilities include an annual SCUBA trip to the Cayman Islands and an annual surf trip to Panama (motorcycle and scooter tours are going to be added soon). Though the trips are drug and alcohol free, Easy Does It welcomes friends and partners who may not be in recovery.

Sobriety Sports Tours: (sobrietysportstours.com)

Sobriety Sports Tours offers unique packages for those looking to combine travel, major sporting events, recovery-based meetings and fellowship into the experience of a lifetime. Scheduling trips around major sports events—such as the Super Bowl, NASCAR races, and their recent East Coast Baseball Tour—Sobriety Sports creates tailored packages for groups of 10-20. They take care of the travel arrangements, hotel accommodations, tickets, local 12-step meetings, and tee times.

Sober Surf Retreats: (oceanasurf.com/travelsober.html)

OceanaSurf offers sober surf trips for those who are interested in keeping clean while riding waves. The trips run periodically throughout the year, all heading to beautiful Baja California Sur in Mexico, and can accommodate small groups of 10 or less. Sober Surf will soon be adding Surf-Yoga Retreats as well as All-Girl Surf Trips to their roster—combining gorgeous accommodations, daily surf instruction, 12-step meetings, and meditation for a surf experience like no other.

Sober Travel Vacations (sobertraveladventures.com)
Alcohol-free vacations for health conscious people who crave adventure one day at a time.

Mental Health

National Institute of Mental Health (http://www.nimh.nih.gov/)
Results of biomedical research on mind and behavior.

National Alliance for the Mentally Ill (http://www.nami.org/)
Support for consumers with mental illness

Substance Abuse & Mental Health Services Administration
(http://www.samhsa.gov/)
United States Department of Health & Human Services

Government Resources

Single-State Agency (SSA) Directory:
(http://www.recoverymonth.gov/Recovery-Month-
Kit/Resources/Single-State-Agency-SSA-Directory.aspx) Prevention
and Treatment of Substance Use and Mental Disorders – A list of State
offices that can provide local information and guidance about
substance use and mental disorders, treatment, and recovery in your
community.

AMVETS (http://www.amvets.org/) This organization provides
support for veterans and the active military in procuring their earned
entitlements. It also offers community services that enhance the quality
of life for this Nation's citizens.

Professionals

Intervention Project for Nurses (http://www.ipnfl.org/)
Help for professionals with chemical dependencies.

International Lawyers in Alcoholics Anonymous (ILAA)
(http://www.ilaa.org/)
This organization serves as a clearinghouse for support groups for lawyers who are recovering from alcohol or other chemical dependencies.

International Pharmacists Anonymous (IPA)
(http://home.comcast.net/~mitchfields/ipa/ipapage.htm)
This is a 12-step fellowship of pharmacists and pharmacy students recovering from any addiction.

Other

This Center for Substance Abuse Prevention widget (http://www.samhsa.gov/about/csap.aspx) includes a variety of updates on activities relating to underage drinking which is updated regularly with local, state, and national articles published by online sources.

NCADD: (http://ncadd.org/) The National Council on Alcoholism and Drug Dependence, Inc. (NCADD) and its Affiliate Network is a voluntary health organization dedicated to fighting the Nation's #1 health problem – alcoholism, drug addiction and the devastating consequences of alcohol and other drugs on individuals, families and communities.

American Council for Drug Education (http://www.acde.org/)
Educational programs and services for teens, parents, and educators

AlcoholScreening.org - Website offering an online screening tool to assess drinking patterns. The website offers visitors free confidential online screenings to assess their drinking patterns, giving them personalized feedback and showing them if their alcohol consumption is likely to be within safe limits. AlcoholScreening.org was developed by Join Together, a project of the Boston University School of Public Health, and was launched in April 2001. The website also provides answers to frequently asked questions about alcohol and health consequences, and provides links to support resources and a database of local treatment programs. Disclaimer: This site does not provide a diagnosis of alcohol abuse, alcohol dependence or any other medical condition. The information provided here cannot substitute for a full evaluation by a health professional, and should only be used as a guide to understanding your alcohol use and the potential health issues involved with it.

About the Author

Taite Adams is a successful marketer and published author who has traded in the high cost of low living for a much more peaceful, and rewarding, life. Free of alcohol and drugs for over a decade and an active member of Alcoholics Anonymous, Taite (not her real name) enjoys living a sober life and sharing those joys with her family, friends and people looking for a better way to live. She is an avid boater, licensed Coast Guard Captain and prolific traveler. While her bucket list remains long, each day brings a shining new opportunity to cross something off the list or discover something new - and for that she remains forever grateful. Check out our active Facebook Page: Taite Adams Recovery Books.

As you begin your Road to Recovery, please check out Taite's other book, Kickstart Your Recovery, available in both Kindle and Paperback.

Should you require additional assistance with your home detox, be sure to pick up Taite's popular book, Safely Detox From Alcohol and Drugs at Home, also on Amazon.com.

Opiate Addiction has reached epidemic proportions in this country and is something that Taite is intimately familiar with. Read her latest book, that is climbing the charts on Amazon, chronicling this insidious killer and laying the pathway for freedom from its grip.

It's hard to miss mention in the media of the drug Molly and the controversy surrounding its use and it's ingredients. There is plenty of confusion there as well. Check out Taite's latest book, called Who is Molly? for the latest info on this drug and its dangers.

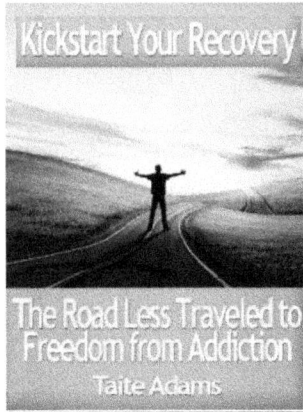

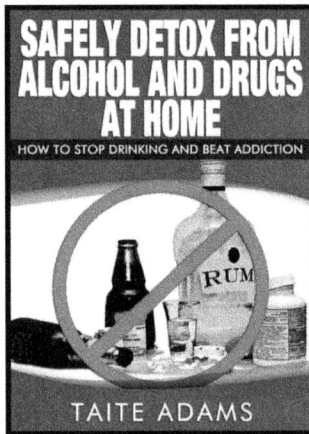

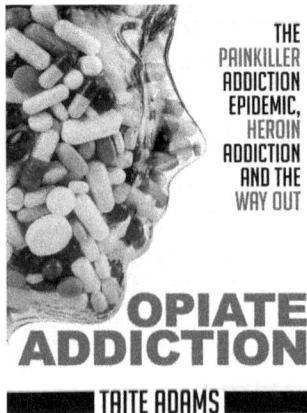

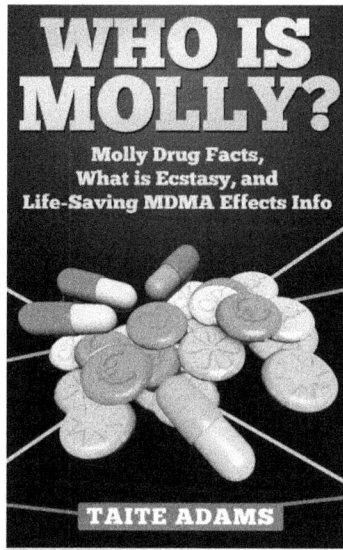

WHO IS MOLLY?

Molly Drug Facts,
What is Ecstasy, and
Life-Saving MDMA Effects Info

TAITE ADAMS

Preface

The world of opiate addiction is ever-changing and has a lot to do with market conditions. Supply and demand and basic economics play a greater role than many people realize in which drugs come in and out of fashion at a particular point in time. Regardless of which form of opiates are popular at the present moment, there is little doubt that opiates will always be one of the most widely abused classes of drugs. Whether it be Vicodin, Oxys, Perc 30s, methadone or heroin, the opiate addict will generally take what they can get their hands on and then abuse the hell out of it.

Opiates have a very long and rich history of being "in fashion", later shunned by society and then finding their medicinal use for the management of pain. It was this rise in the use of prescription opiate painkillers, however, that has brought about what the CDC is now calling an epidemic of prescription drug addiction. In fact, in 2011 nearly 1.8 million Americans were addicted to some form of prescription painkiller, more than those addicted to cocaine and heroin combined. I had already been clean from my opiate addiction for over 10 years by this time, yet the memory of the day to day struggle, the terror and hopelessness are still fresh in my mind. This is not something that I expect to ever forget and it was interesting to re-live some of it and learn a few new "tricks" in the writing of this book.

What scares the hell out of me more than anything else is the rising problem, in epidemic proportions, of heroin use in this country as a direct result of prescription opiate addiction. There is no doubt that prescription painkillers serve as a gateway to heroin use and this is deadly. While abuse of prescription pills for pain was reported to be going down in 2011, according to the national survey on drug use and health, heroin use was reported to be increasing. In fact, in 2011, nearly 200,000 people tried heroin for the first time. In 2014, it's use and abuse is nearly out of control.

If you or a loved one are addicted to opiates, this book is for you. In it you can learn more about the drugs that you have been taking, their effects on your body and mind and what you can do to break free. There is information on opiate maintenance programs as well as warnings on their long-term use and some good information about opiate detox and making treatment center decisions. Recovery from opiate addiction isn't easy but it is absolutely possible and I have found that it is infinitely simpler and more fulfilling than that of the day to day life of a hopeless opiate addict.

Taite Adams

The Opiate Addiction Epidemic

Nobody will laugh long who deals much with opium: its pleasures even are of a grave and solemn complexion. -Thomas de Quincey

Most people think that they have a clear picture in their mind of what a drug addict is but generally, when it comes to opiate addiction, what you get couldn't be further from that image. Opiate addicts do not fit a general stereotype as the drug does not discriminate. Because of the nature of opiate addiction, it strikes across age, ethnic and economic groups and then pulls each and every one of those stricken down with equal measure.

The CDC recently reported that opiate addiction is now America's fastest growing drug problem, with the total number of painkillers prescribed in a single year enough to medicate every adult living in the U.S. around the clock. While true that heroin is the most widely used illegal opiate, it's a fact that prescription opiate painkillers are equally dangerous and an insidious problem. The World Health Organization (WHO) estimates that approximately two million people in the United States alone are addicted to prescription opiates.

The problem is also not limited to adults, as first use of opiates seems to be getting younger. The National Institute on Drug Abuse (NIDA) reports that an estimated 52 million people, 20% of those aged 12 and older, have used prescription drugs for nonmedical reasons at least once. Also, about 1 in 12 high school seniors reported nonmedical use of the prescription drug Vicodin the past year. About

1 in 20 high school seniors also reported abusing OxyContin. This isn't limited to the younger crowd either. According to a 2011 study by the Substance Abuse and Mental Health Services Administration (SAMHSA), the rate of current illicit drug use in adults aged 50 to 59 increased to 6.3% in 2011 from 2.7% in 2002 with opiates being among the most commonly abused drugs. The total number of opiate prescriptions dispensed by retail pharmacies in the United States rose from 76 million in 1991 to 210 million in 2010.

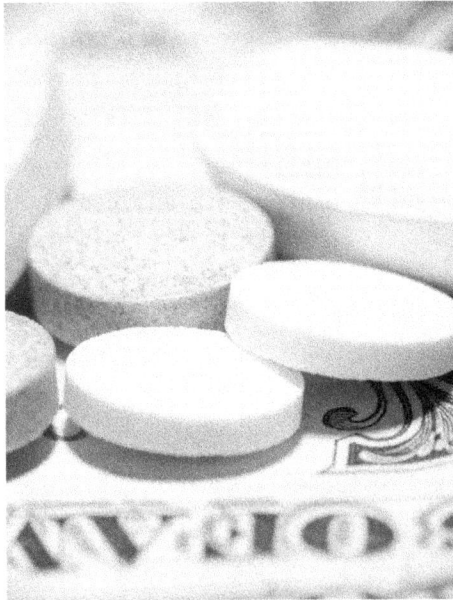

The epidemic of opiate addiction and painkiller addiction has resulted in nearly 16,000 overdose deaths annually. While heroin continues to be a rising problem, opiate addiction in general is not the stereotypical drug problem that many of us think of when we picture the "war on drugs". In fact, many times this involves a patient who began with a legitimate pain issue, an unwitting string of physicians (or not) who are writing these prescriptions, and pharmaceutical companies who are acting within the law. The public consumption of opiates, through legal channels, is costing health insurers over \$72 billion annually.

Opiates are a huge problem! ...and growing. Trust me, I know. Most of the time we start taking them for a legitimate pain issue, whether for a root canal or some major surgery. Many times the addiction to them develops over a period of time as a physical dependency develops. With others, however, there is an instantaneous "pull" that these drugs have on you because of the way that they make you feel. They not only take away the physical pain that they were prescribed for, but bring to the table something that you thought you had been looking for for a very long time. This is how it was for me. Those pills became my best friend and my salvation for a time - until they completely owned me.

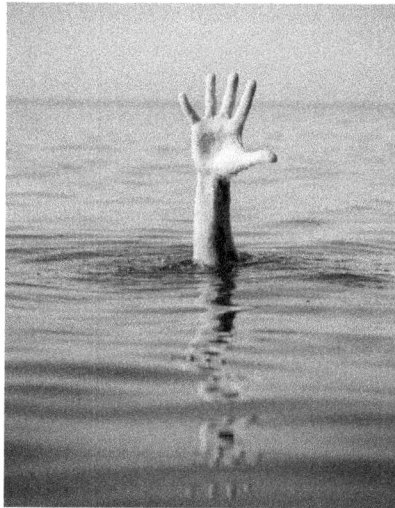

Restart Your Recovery

You will find peace not by trying to escape your problems, but by confronting them courageously. You will find peace not in denial, but in victory. -J. Donald Walters

...keep reading *HERE* --> **Get more information at** **www.TaiteAdams.com**

Taite Adams